Emergency Room Orthopaedic Procedures
An Illustrative Guide for the House Officer

Emergency Room Orthopaedic Procedures
An Illustrative Guide for the House Officer

Kenneth A Egol MD
Professor and Vice Chairman
Department of Orthopaedic Surgery
New York University Hospital for Joint Diseases, NY

Eric J Strauss MD
Assistant Professor
Department of Orthopaedic Surgery
New York University Hospital for Joint Diseases, NY

Foreword
Joseph D Zuckerman, MD

JAYPEE BROTHERS MEDICAL PUBLISHERS (P) LTD

New Delhi • Panama City • London

Jaypee Brothers Medical Publishers (P) Ltd.

Headquarter

Jaypee Brothers Medical Publishers (P) Ltd
4838/24, Ansari Road, Daryaganj
New Delhi 110 002, India
Phone: +91-11-43574357
Fax: +91-11-43574314
Email: jaypee@jaypeebrothers.com

Overseas Offices

J.P. Medical Ltd.,
83 Victoria Street London
SW1H 0HW (UK)
Phone: +44-2031708910
Fax: +02-03-0086180
Email: info@jpmedpub.com

Jaypee-Highlights Medical Publishers Inc.
City of Knowledge, Bld. 237, Clayton
Panama City, Panama
Phone: +50-73-010496
Fax: +50-73-010499
Email: cservice@jphmedical.com

Website: www.jaypeebrothers.com
Website: www.jaypeedigital.com

Inquiries for bulk sales may be solicited at: jaypee@jaypeebrothers.com

This book has been published in good faith that the contents provided by the author(s) contained herein are original, and is intended for educational purposes only. While every effort is made to ensure the accuracy of information, the publisher and the author(s) specifically disclaim any damage, liability, or loss incurred, directly or indirectly, from the use or application of any of the contents of this work. If not specifically stated, all figures and tables are courtesy of the author(s). Where appropriate, the readers should consult with a specialist or contact the manufacturer of the drug or device.

Emergency Room Orthopaedic Procedures: An Illustrative Guide for the House Officer
First Edition: **2012**

ISBN 978-93-5025-570-4

Printed at Replika Press Pvt. Ltd.

Dedication

I dedicate this book to my family, Lori, Alex, Jonathan and Gabby for their unending support and to all those who dedicate themselves to train the physicians of the future.

—Kenneth A Egol

This book is dedicated to my wife Stacey and son Jacob for their continued love and support.

—Eric J Strauss

Contributors

Colin Prensky MD
Research Associate
Department of Orthopaedic
Surgery
New York University Hospital for
Joint Diseases, NY

Eric J Strauss MD
Assistant Professor
Department of Orthopaedic
Surgery
New York University Hospital
for Joint Diseases, NY

Kenneth A Egol MD
Professor and Vice Chairman
Department of Orthopaedic
Surgery
New York University Hospital
for Joint Diseases, NY

Robert C Rothberg
Associate Professor
Department of Emergency
Medicine
New York University Hospital for
Joint Diseases, NY

Sonya Khurana MD
Research Associate
Department of Orthopaedic
Surgery
New York University Hospital for
Joint Diseases, NY

Foreword

Orthopaedic injuries and disorders are a very common reason for patients to visit emergency rooms in the United States. In 2008, over 7 million individuals presented to emergency rooms in the United States with a principle or primary diagnosis related to the musculoskeletal system. (1) When all secondary diagnoses are considered, this number increased to almost 23 million. (2) Clearly, a significant amount of care for musculoskeletal conditions is provided in the emergency department setting. Therefore, the more knowledgeable and experienced emergency room physicians become in the evaluation and treatment of musculoskeletal injuries and disorders, the higher the quality of care that can be provided. In this context, this is a very important – in fact, essential – textbook. Dr Egol and Dr Strauss have prepared a "How To Guide" for diagnosis and treatment of common musculoskeletal injuries. The text combines photographs, illustrations and step by step instructions and demonstrate how to perform essential interventions needed in the emergency department for the management of orthopaedic injuries. It will be essential reading for emergency room physicians, residents, students and staff.

Dr Egol and Dr Strauss are the perfect authors for this textbook. Their experience, expertise and commitment to education at all levels is well-recognized by their peers. This textbook reflects the teaching that they do each and every day and have been doing throughout their careers. In the past, this has primarily benefitted the faculty, housestaff and students at the Hospital for Joint Diseases and NYU Langone Medical Center. With the publication of this textbook, it will now benefit thousands of other healthcare professionals providing emergency care for musculoskeletal injuries and disorders. As a result, patients will be better cared with the potential for improved outcome. For this we owe Dr Egol and Dr Strauss both our respect and gratitude.

Joseph D Zuckerman, MD
Professor and Chair
NYU Hospital for Joint Diseases
Department of Orthopaedic Surgery

HCU Pret, Healthcare Cost and Utilization Project: Agency for Healthcare, Research and Quality, Rockville, MD; http://hcupnet.ahrg.gov

National Center for Health Statistics: National Ambulatory Medical Care Survey (NHAMCS), Hyattsville, MD: Public Health Service, 2008.

Preface

The idea for this book arose from the countless hours that we have spent training orthopaedic surgery residents at the NYU Hospital for Joint Diseases. During the course of teaching a new crop of orthopaedic residents the basics of many of the orthopaedic procedures we perform in the emergency department setting; it became clear to us that no text was available to aid in the process. The majority of this type of teaching has been provided by senior residents who instruct their junior residents on how to perform joint and fracture reductions, compartment measurements, joint aspirations, nail-bed repairs and simple laceration treatment. While this type of knowledge, handed down from one generation to the next generation of resident has been adequate, we felt that a step by step manual with easy to follow directions, including the materials needed and techniques utilized to perform each procedure was warranted and would be a useful reference for treating orthopaedic pathology in the emergency room.

This manual has been prepared in a manner that will aid any house officer in any discipline, as well as any healthcare provider who is charged with attending to patients presenting to the emergency department with an acute traumatic musculoskeletal complaint in need of intervention. Despite the ever-increasing expanse of knowledge within the medical field, this text focuses on the basics of urgent orthopaedic procedural care. This first edition, pocket sized guide contains the necessary information needed to perform the procedures described here within. We hope that the users of this text find it useful in their daily care of patients with musculoskeletal complaints.

Kenneth A Egol MD
Eric J Strauss MD

Contents

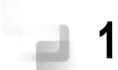

1

Nerve Blocks Around the Hand

Sonya Khurana, Kenneth A Egol

INTRODUCTION

Digital nerve blocks provide regional anesthesia for procedures performed on the fingers. Other options for anesthesia around the hand include local injections and topical creams. However, due to the sensitivity of the palmar surface, local injection may be quite painful and ineffective as compared to a nerve block. Digital nerve blocks anesthetize a larger area, usually utilize a lesser amount of anesthetic, and prevent further distortion of the injured tissues as compared to local injection. However, the onset is usually several minutes and they are more technically challenging to perform. Accidental injection into a systemic blood vessel can also occur and the injection site may become very tense and thus potentially compromise digital perfusion.

Each digit is innervated by two digital nerves that arise from the median or ulnar nerve. In order to perform surgery on the digit, both nerves must be blocked. Sensation to the dorsal aspect of the digit is provided by branches of the digital nerves that course dorsally at each joint. By using a digital nerve block, adequate anesthesia can be obtained for all procedures distal to the proximal phalanx. For more proximal anesthesia, a wrist block is more effective. For procedures on the dorsal aspect of the hand and up to the skin on the dorsum of the proximal phalanx, a nerve block involving the superficial branch of the radial nerve and/or dorsal branch of the ulnar nerve will be necessary. Digital blood vessels run along the flexor tendon sheath with the nerves.

Indications for digital nerve blocks include lacerations beyond the mid-proximal phalanx, nail bed injuries, foreign bodies in the digit, finger fractures and finger and/or nail bed infection. Contraindications include infection of the tissues through which the needle will pass, compromised blood supply and an allergy to the anesthetic. Epinephrine should not be used for digital nerve blocks, especially in patients at risk for digit infarction or ischemia, such as those with peripheral vascular disease or diabetes mellitus. Epinephrine causes the blood vessels to constrict and should be avoided secondary to the proximity of the digital arteries to the digital nerves.

There are several techniques utilized when performing digital nerve blocks. According to a meta-analysis and trial performed by Yin et al. Single subcutaneous palmar injection digital blocks were equally painful to traditional digital blocks. Transthecal blocks were found to be more painful than the other two. This may be because in the latter technique, the anesthetic is inserted into the flexor tendon sheath, which has little space, thus producing higher hydraulic pressure and increasing the pain. A drawback to the palmar block technique is potentially inadequate anesthesia of the dorsum of the digit because the dorsal sensory nerves may not always be blocked.

Advantages to the transthecal digital block include a single injection that anesthetizes the entire digit, less anesthetic, rapid onset of anesthesia and little risk of trauma to the neurovascular bundles. Disadvantages include increased pain even after the anesthetic wears off and a more technically challenging procedure. Additionally, it is important to use sterile technique for this procedure, due to consequences of infection in the flexor tendon sheath.

Wrist blocks can be performed instead of digital blocks when the area in a particular nerve distribution needs to be anesthetized. Indications for wrist blocks include multiple finger fractures, finger/nail bed lacerations, reduction of metacarpal shaft or neck fractures. Contraindications are the same as those for digital nerve blocks.

The three nerves that pass through the wrist, the ulnar, median and radial nerves, play an important role in nerve blocks around the hand (Figs 1.1 and 1.2). The ulnar nerve travels through Guyon's canal, which is formed by the pisiform and hamate carpal bones and the pisohamate ligament. The canal begins at the proximal end of the transverse carpal ligament and ends at the aponeurotic arch of

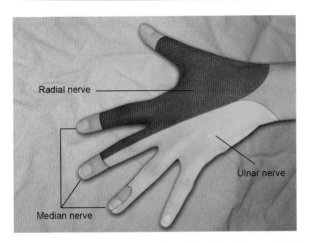

Fig. 1.1 Sensory dermatomal distribution of the dorsal aspect of the hand

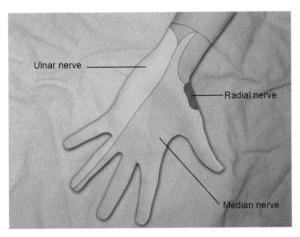

Fig. 1.2 Sensory dermatomal distribution of the palmar aspect of the hand

the hypothenar muscles. The nerve provides sensation to the little finger and the ulnar side of the ring finger and motor function to the intrinsic muscles. The dorsal branch of the ulnar nerve arises 5 to 8 cm proximal to Guyon's canal and travels in a dorsal-ulnar direction to provide sensation to the dorsal-ulnar aspect of the hand and the medial 1.5 digits up to the MP joint level. The median nerve passes through the carpal tunnel, which lies deep to the palmaris longus. It is bordered proximally by the pisiform and tubercle of the scaphoid, distally by the hook of the hamate and the tubercle of the trapezium, laterally by the scaphoid and trapezium, medially by the hamate and pisiform, and superiorly by the transverse carpal ligament. The median nerve supplies sensation to the palmar aspect of radial 3.5 digits and the thenar eminence (the terminal branches of the lateral antebrachial cutaneous nerve may also provide sensory coverage as distal as the thenar crease). The palmar cutaneous branch of the median nerve arises 5 to 8 cm proximal to the carpal canal and provides sensation to the palmar skin up to the MP joint level. The superficial branch of the radial nerve wraps around the distal portion of the radius toward the dorsal aspect of the hand. It gives sensation to the dorsal-radial aspect of the hand and the dorsum of the lateral three digits up to the MCP joints.

Indications for median nerve blocks are multiple finger fractures and finger/nailbed lacerations. Indications for ulnar nerve blocks include ulnar-sided lacerations and reduction of boxer's fracture if anesthesia is required. Radial nerve blocks are used when there are lacerations on thumb and dorsum of hand.

MATERIALS

A 10 ml syringe with 18 to 22-gauge needle for drawing up anesthetic, local anesthetic (such as lidocaine 1%) without epinephrine and buffered with a 1:10 ratio of sodium bicarbonate 8.4 percent, 27 to 30-gauge needle for performing the injection.

STEPS

For any technique, thoroughly prepare the area to be injected and/ or sutured with alcohol, iodine or chlorhexidine prior to injection.

■ Step 1: Finger Web Space Block

- Pronate the patient's hand and place flat on a sterile drape. The dorsum of the hand is less sensitive to pain than the palmar aspect.
- Insert the needle perpendicular to the finger and into the subcutaneous tissue of the web space just distal to the MCP joint (Figs 1.3A and B).
- Slowly aspirate to ensure that the needle is not in a digital blood vessel.

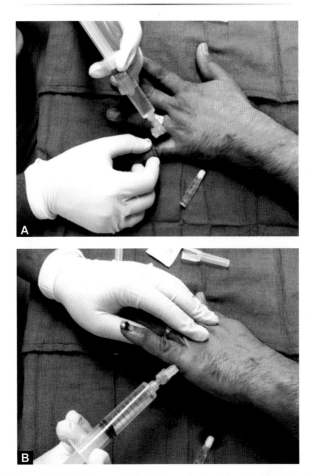

Figs 1.3A and B Digital nerve block is performed by injecting local anesthetic perpendicular to the finger both medially and laterally to anesthetize the radial and ulnar digital nerves

- Inject 2 ml of anesthetic into the subcutaneous dorsal tissue, infiltrating the tissues around the dorsal nerve.
- Slowly advance the needle towards the palmar surface and inject an additional 2 ml of anesthetic as the needle goes along. This should infiltrate the tissues surrounding the palmar nerve. Do not push through the palmar skin surface.
- Withdraw the needle and repeat these steps on the opposite side of the finger. Use 2 ml of anesthetic per nerve (for 8 ml total).

- Do not connect the bridge dorsally, it is important not to create a ring block by infiltrating the anesthetic in a circumferential manner as this can compromise the blood supply.

Step 2: Transthecal Technique (Through Flexor Tendon Sheath)

- Palpate the distal palmar crease and flex the digit to help identify the flexor tendon.
- Supinate the patient's hand and place flat on a sterile drape.
- Insert the needle (without the syringe attached) at a 45° angle and penetrate the skin surface just distal to the distal palmar crease.
- Advance the needle into the flexor tendon sheath.
- In order to confirm placement of the needle, passively flex and extend the finger. If the needle is in the sheath, it should swing in an arc with tendon movement.
- Attach the syringe and slowly inject the anesthetic (2 ml). The anesthetic should flow easily into the tendon sheath.

Step 3: Wrist Block-Median Nerve

- Supinate the forearm and place on a sterile drape. Place the needle between the palmaris longus and flexor carpi radialis tendons, about 2 cm proximal to the wrist flexion crease (Fig. 1.4).

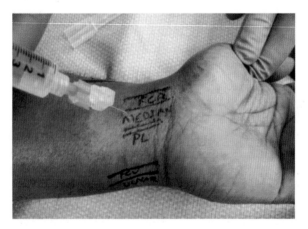

Fig. 1.4 Median nerve block performed by injecting local anesthetic between the palmaris longus and flexor carpi radialis tendons

- The needle should be inserted at a 45° angle and penetrate about 1.5 cm into the underlying tissue. Slowly start to inject 5 to 7 cc of anesthetic into the area. If the patient reports an immediate feeling of electric sensation, this could indicate that the needle has penetrated the nerve. Withdraw the needle slightly and continue. Direct injection into the nerve is painful and should be avoided.

- The final 3 cc of anesthetic can be injected in the subcutaneous tissues in a radial direction from the palmaris longus, just radial to the flexor carpi radialis. This will anesthetize the palmar cutaneous portion of the median nerve and improve the quality of the block for procedures that require a palmar skin incision (carpal tunnel release).

■ Step 4: Wrist Block-Ulnar Nerve

- Supinate the hand and place it on a sterile drape.
- Insert the needle 6 cm proximal to the wrist crease, and ulnar and dorsal to the flexor carpi ulnaris in a transverse manner (Figs 1.5A and B). If the needle is placed more distally, it will miss the dorsal branch of the ulnar nerve, which can be blocked by a subcutaneous wheal placed between the ulnar styloid and the pisiform on the ulnar aspect of the wrist.
- Inject 8 to 10 ml of anesthetic.

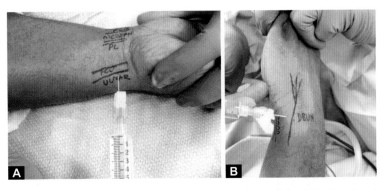

Figs 1.5A and B (A) Ulnar nerve block performed by injecting local anesthe–tic proximal to the wrist flexion crease, dorsal and ulnar to the flexor carpi ulnaris tendon; (B) The dorsal branch of the ulnar nerve is also blocked by injecting local anesthetic dorsal to the ulnar styloid

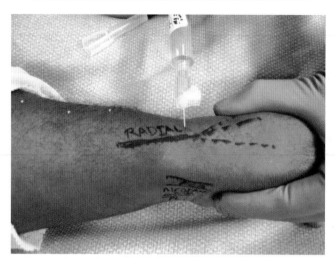

Fig. 1.6 Superficial radial nerve block performed by injecting local anesthetic 2 cm proximal to the tip of the radial styloid along the radial aspect of the distal forearm

■ Step 5: Wrist Block-Radial Nerve

- Pronate the hand and place it on a sterile drape.
- Insert the needle 2 cm proximal to the tip of the radial styloid along the radial aspect of the distal forearm (Fig. 1.6). Inject 7 to 10 cc of anesthetic along the radial and dorsal aspect of the wrist and distal forearm, between the first and third dorsal compartments (the tendons of the abductor pollicis longus, and extensor pollicis brevis and the extensor pollicis longus).

SUGGESTED READINGS

1. Chale S, Singer AJ, Marchini S, et al. Digital versus local anesthesia for finger lacerations: A randomized controlled trial. Academic Emergency Medicine. 2006;13(10):1046-50.
2. Chiu DT. Transthecal digital block: Flexor tendon sheath used for anesthetic infusion. J Hand Surg Am. 1990;15(3):471-3.4.
3. Egol Kenneth A, Kenneth J Koval, Joseph D Zuckerman. Handbook of Fractures, 4th edn. Philadelphia, PA: Lippincott Williams & Wilkins; 2010. pp. 68-9.

4. Setnik and Thomson Associates. Local anesthesia techniques [online]. The Multimedia Procedure Manual. Available from http://emprocedures.com/anesthesia/pharmacology.htm
5. Whetzel TP, Mabourakh S, Barkhordar R. Modified transthecal digital block. J Hand Surg Am. 1997;22(2):361-3.
6. Yin ZG, Zhang JB, Kan SL, et al. A comparison of traditional digital blocks and single subcutaneous palmar injection blocks at the base of the finger and a meta-analysis of the digital block trials. Journal of Hand Surgery (British and European Volume). 2006;31(5):547-55.

2

The Evaluation and Management of Ankle Fractures: Reduction and Splinting Techniques

Eric J Strauss

INTRODUCTION

Ankle fractures, commonly present to the emergency department, following injuries sustained during athletic participation or from higher energy traumatic events. They account for 12 percent of all bony injuries and often are the result of a rotational mechanism. Important factors influencing the type of ankle fracture sustained include the patient's age, bone quality, position of the foot at the time of injury, and the magnitude, direction and rate of the force applied. The following chapter will review the relevant anatomy, methods of evaluation, classification and techniques for both fracture reduction and splinting.

RELEVANT ANATOMY

The ankle is a hinge or saddle-type joint, composed of the distal tibia, the distal fibula and the dome of the talus. The articular surface of the distal tibia (the plafond) combined with the medial and lateral malleoli form the ankle mortise, which is a constrained articulation for the talar dome. The dome of the talus is approximately 2.5 mm wider anteriorly than it is posteriorly, helping provide ankle stability in the dorsiflexed position during weight-bearing activities.

The ankle is supported by a system of ligamentous structures including the anterior talofibular ligament (ATFL), posterior talofibular ligament (PTFL) and calcaneofibular ligament (CFL) laterally, and the deltoid ligament complex medially (composed of a superficial portion and a deep intra-articular portion). Additional support is provided by the syndesmotic ligament complex, which provides resistance to rotational, axial and translational forces by connecting the distal tibia and fibula (Fig. 2.1). The syndesmosis is comprised of the anterior inferior tibiofibular ligament (AITFL), the posterior inferior tibiofibular ligament (PITFL), the transverse tibiofibular ligament and the interosseous ligament which is a distal extension of the syndesmotic membrane.

Functionally, ankle motion occurs in dorsiflexion and plantar flexion, with 30° of dorsiflexion and 45° of plantar flexion, is considered normal. Inversion and eversion of the ankle takes place at the level of the subtalar joint, formed at the articulation of the talus and the calcaneus. Secondary to the strength of the ligamentous structures supporting the subtalar joint, inversion and eversion forces tend to cause injury to the structural components of the ankle joint.

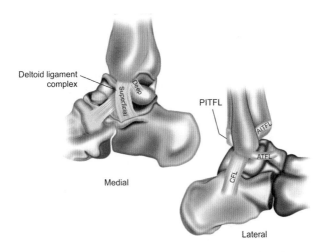

Fig. 2.1 The ankle joint is stabilized by its supporting ligaments including the anterior talofibular ligament (ATFL), posterior talofibular ligament (PTFL) and calcaneofibular ligament (CFL) laterally and the deltoid ligament complex medially.

PRESENTATION AND EVALUATION IN THE EMERGENCY ROOM

Patients with ankle fractures typically present to the ER with complaints of pain, swelling and difficulty with weightbearing activities following a rotational type mechanism of injury (Fig. 2.2). They may have gross deformity present which should alert the evaluating physician to the possibility of a fracture dislocation. Some patients may be capable of weightbearing with discomfort despite the presence of bony injury while others may be unable to bear any weight at all on the injured lower extremity.

The initial evaluation includes an inspection of the injured ankle, noting the presence of deformity and the condition of the surrounding soft tissue, looking for evidence of an open injury or the presence of blistering.

A careful neurovascular examination should be performed and documented in the patient's chart. Next, the entire length of the fibula should be palpated for tenderness and the presence of a bony step-off, indicative of a displaced fracture. Palpation of the ankle should

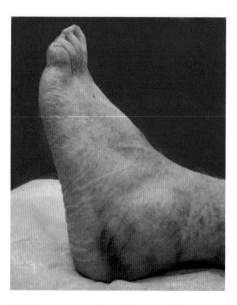

Fig. 2.2 Patient who presented to the emergency room with a left ankle fracture. Note the ecchymosis and swelling present about the lateral aspect of the ankle in the region of the lateral malleolus

be continued medially, looking for tenderness over the medial malleolus and the deltoid ligament complex. A "squeeze test" can then be performed by squeezing 5 cm proximal to the intermalleolar line to identify a possible injury to the syndesmosis.

RADIOGRAPHIC EVALUATION

A three-view series of the ankle is typically utilized for the diagnosis of ankle fractures in the ER. This series is composed of an anteroposterior (AP) view, a lateral view and a mortise view (Figs 2.3A-C).

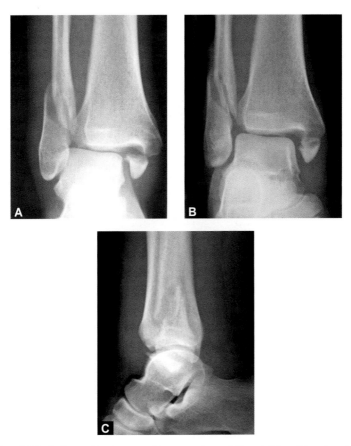

Figs 2.3A-C An ankle trauma X-ray series of the right ankle showing evidence of displaced bimalleolar ankle fracture (A) Anteroposterior; (B) Mortise; (C) Lateral

The mortise view is taken as an anteroposterior view with the foot internally rotated 15 to 20° such that the beam is perpendicular to the intermalleolar axis providing a clear view of the articulations between the plafond, the lateral malleolus and the talar dome.

The Ottawa ankle rules were developed to help predict which ankle injuries were likely fractures and guide the treating physician as to when ankle X-rays are appropriate (Fig. 2.4).

Validated in a number of clinical studies including a meta-analysis, the Ottawa ankle rules have been demonstrated to have a sensitivity nearing 100 precent coupled with a 30 to 40 percent reduction in the number of X-rays taken.

When appropriately indicated, the three-view ankle series can be evaluated for the evidence of fracture lines, fracture fragment displacement, abnormal relationships between the bony components of the joint, and fracture classification by both location and pattern. The AP and mortise views can be evaluated for normal relationships between the components of the ankle joint including the extent of tibiofibular overlap, tibiofibular clear space, talar tilt, the amount of medial clear space present, the talocrural angle and the extent of talar shift that is present.

Advanced imaging in the form of CT scans or MRI is typically not required in the workup of a rotational ankle fracture. A CT scan may

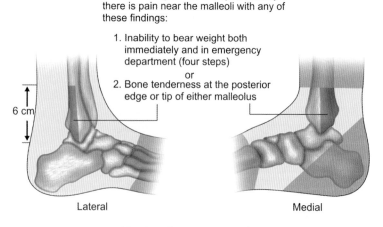

An ankle X-ray series is only necessary if there is pain near the malleoli with any of these findings:

1. Inability to bear weight both immediately and in emergency department (four steps)
   or
2. Bone tenderness at the posterior edge or tip of either malleolus

6 cm

Lateral

Medial

Fig. 2.4 Ottawa ankle rules
Source: Reprint from JAMA. 1993;269:1127

however be useful in evaluating a pediatric patient with a suspected triplane fracture or in the case of a complex, comminuted fracture to help identify fracture fragments.

Stress views of the ankle may be indicated in an effort to differentiate between a supination-external rotation Type II or III injury which can be managed nonoperatively and a supination-external rotation Type IV equivalent injury which is unstable and requires operative fixation. A stress view is performed as a mortise view with the examiner applying an external rotation force to the foot as the X-ray is taken (Figs 2.5A and B).

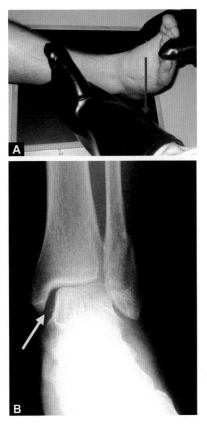

Figs 2.5A and B (A) Application of external rotation force during a stress radiograph of the right ankle. The red arrow shows the direction of the applied stress; (B) The stress radiograph is examined for evidence of medial clear space widening as is shown with the yellow arrow

The examiner should be protected in a lead apron with lead gloves during this procedure. An increase in the amount of medial clear space on the mortise view (>5 millimeters) with applied stress is an indicator of injury to the deltoid ligament complex and thus an unstable injury. A gravity stress view can also be utilized.

ANKLE FRACTURE REDUCTION

Proper closed reduction of a displaced, unstable ankle fracture is of paramount importance in an effort to prevent further injury to the articular surfaces of the talus and plafond, prevent pressure injury to the overlying skin and subcutaneous tissue and help to facilitate a more rapid resolution of the soft-tissue swelling associated with the injury. The goals of a closed reduction are restoration of the anatomic mortise with the talar dome centered underneath the tibial plafond. The reduction maneuver will be followed by splint immobilization, so any open wounds or injury-associated blisters should be addressed before reduction is attempted.

In most cases, ankle fracture reduction will involve applying a force in the direction opposite to that which caused the injury (i.e. applying a pronation-internal rotation force to a supination-external rotation type fracture pattern).

- Typically for the reduction, the patient is supine on the stretcher and the injured leg is either supported by an assistant or the patient is positioned such that the injured ankle is off the end of the bed, providing adequate access.
- It is often beneficial to provide the patient with pain medication prior to reduction to make the process more tolerable. Based on the appearance of the X-ray, a manual force will be applied to reduce the talus back into position.
- As an example, for a displaced supination-external (SE) IV ankle fracture, one of the treating physician's hands will be placed on the medial aspect of the patient's lower leg to provide a counterforce while the other provides a medially directed translation force to the lateral aspect of the patient's ankle. Often the talus can be felt to move back into anatomic position.
- The initial steps of splint application are then performed and once the cotton undercast padding (webril) layer has been placed, a second (usually less forceful) reduction maneuver is performed. The cotton undercast padding layer tends to have "memory" which will help to keep the talus reduced as the splint is applied.

For very unstable fractures, Quigley's traction can be applied to help, achieve and maintain reduction as the splint is applied (Fig. 2.6).

- For Quigley's traction, a long piece of 6-inch stockinette is placed on the injured lower extremity and pulled up to the level of the proximal thigh.
- The proximal end of the stockinette is either held by the patient or clamped into place to provide traction.
- The distal end of the stockinette is then brought over the contra-lateral shoulder applying a pronation and internal rotation force to the injured ankle.
- Under appropriate tension, the distal end of the stockinette is tied to the IV pole on the stretcher. A manual reduction maneuver can be used to supplement that achieved with Quigley's traction (Fig. 2.7).

■ Splint Application

Following reduction of a displaced fracture, a plaster posterior splint with a U-shaped component is applied to immobilize the ankle. This is typically performed using 4-inch plaster rolls but different size plaster may be necessary depending on patient size.

Materials

Materials required are rolls of plaster, rolls of cotton undercast padding, a basin of lukewarm water and ACE bandages (Fig. 2. 8).

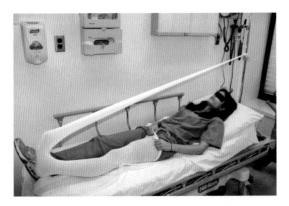

Fig. 2.6 Quigley's traction can help achieve and maintain a reduction for unstable ankle fractures

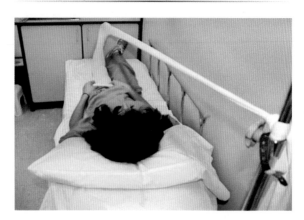

Fig. 2.7 When applying Quigley's traction, the end of the stockinette is tied to the IV pole on the stretcher over the patient's contralateral shoulder

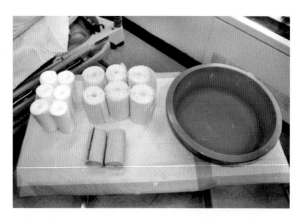

Fig. 2.8 Required materials for splint application include 4 inch plaster, 4 inch cotton undercast padding, 4 inch ACE bandages and a basin of lukewarm water

- Each component of the splint is rolled out to be 8 to 10 layers in thickness, sized in length appropriately such that the posterior component extends from the just distal to the patient's toes to the proximal calf (2–3 fingerbreadths distal to the knee flexion crease to prevent posterior irritation) and the "U" component sized to reach the same level (Figs 2.9A and B).

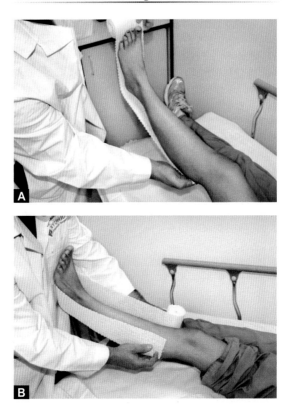

Figs 2.9A and B The length of the posterior and U portions of the splint are measured relative to the size of the patient's lower leg

- To protect the underlying soft tissues, 2 to 3 layers of cotton undercast padding (webril) are applied, making sure no creases or folds are present as this will irritate the skin and can cause pressure injury under the splint (Fig. 2.10).
- The posterior component of the splint is dipped in room temperature and the water is subsequently worked out of the material.
- The posterior component is then placed over the cotton undercast padding layer and molded to the shape of the patient's calf.
- The posterior component is held in place by wrapping a single layer of cotton undercast padding around it.
- The same process is then performed for the "U" component, molding it to the contours of the patient's lower leg once it is applied, especially in the supramalleolar region.

- Once both the components of the splint are in place, they are overwrapped with an ACE bandage (Figs 2.11 and 2.12).
- As the plaster is hardening, the treating physician applies manual force in the direction of the reduction maneuver to facilitate keeping the talus underneath the plafond.
- Additionally, it is important to pay attention to the position of the foot as the reduction is being held. The ankle should be dorsiflexed up into the neutral position which places the wider anterior portion of the talar dome underneath the plafond producing a more stable reduction.

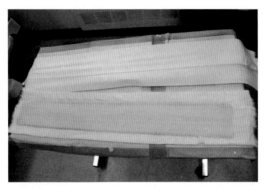

Fig. 2.10 The posterior and U components of the splint are dipped into the lukewarm water and layed on top of a layer of cotton undercast padding

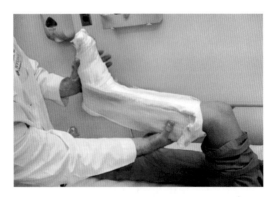

Fig. 2.11 The posterior component is applied first, followed by the U component of the splint

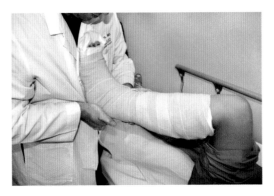

Fig. 2.12 The splint is overwrapped with ACE bandages and the treating practitioner applies a manual reduction force to the ankle. Note the use of the practitioner's chest to maintain the ankle in a neutral position as the plaster dries and hardens

- To facilitate a neutral ankle position, the patient's knee can be flexed to help take tension-off of the gastrocnemius-soleus complex. A commonly used technique at our institution is for the treating physician to place the plantar aspect of the patient's foot (the bottom of the splint) against their chest as the reduction maneuver is being held. This allows the ankle to be held in neutral position as the knee is flexed (Figs 2.13A and B).
- An alternative approach which can be effective especially when an assistant is not available or for fracture patterns that either do not require a manual reduction or one in which only a mild amount of force is expected to be required, is to position the patient prone on the stretcher with the knee flexed to 90°. This give excellent access to the ankle, allows for easy splint application, and facilitates splinting the ankle in a neutral position (Figs 2.14A to D).
- Patients whose reduction is performed using Quigley's traction as an aid can have their splint applied while the traction is held in place. Once the splint has hardened, the stockinette can be cut at both the proximal and distal aspects of the splint.

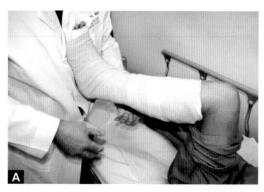

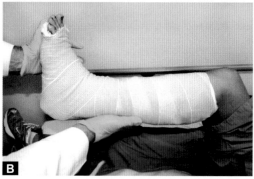

Figs 2.13A and B Knee in the position of flexion to
facilitate neutral ankle position

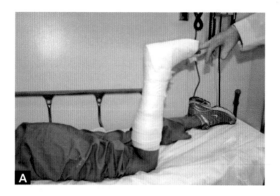

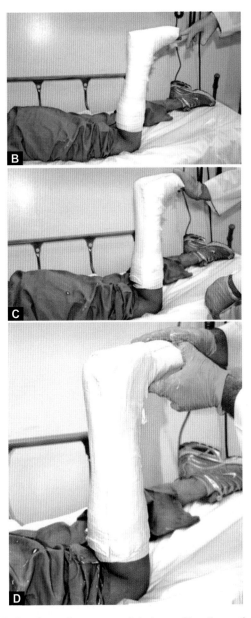

Figs 2.14A-D An alternative approach is to position the patient prone on the stretcher with their knee flexed 90 degrees providing easy access to the ankle for reduction and splint application

POST-REDUCTION CARE

Once the splint has hardened, the patient should be sent for a repeated three-view ankle trauma series to confirm adequate reduction of the fracture. If the talus is adequately reduced under the plafond, the patient is instructed to keep the injured lower extremity elevated with or without the use of ice over the anterior aspect of the splint to help facilitate swelling reduction. They are made non weightbearing using crutches for ambulatory assistance.

SUGGESTED READINGS

■ Textbook Chapters

1. Marsh JL, Saltzman Charles. "Ankle fractures". Rockwood and Green's Fractures in Adults. Chapter 42:2001-91.

■ Review Articles

1. Michelson JD. Ankle fractures resulting from rotational injuries. J Am Acad Orthop Surg. 2003;11:403-12.
2. Zalavras C, Thordarson D. Ankle syndesmotic injury. J Am Acad Orthop Surg. 2007;15:330-39.
3. Van den Bekerom MP, Haverkamp D, Kloen P. Biomechanical and clinical evaluation of posterior malleolar fractures. A systematic review of the literature. J Trauma. 2009;66(1):279-84. Review.

■ Relevant Studies

1. Egol KA, Amirtharajah M, Tejwani NC, et al. Ankle stress test for predicting the need for surgical fixation of isolated fibular fractures. J Bone Joint Surg Am. 2004;86-A(11):2393-8. Erratum in: J Bone Joint Surg Am. 2005;87(4):857. J Bone Joint Surg Am. 2005;87-A(1):161.
2. Egol KA, Tejwani NC, Walsh MG, et al. Predictors of short-term functional outcome following ankle fracture surgery. J Bone Joint Surg Am. 2006;88(5):974-9.
3. Tejwani NC, McLaurin TM, Walsh M, et al. Are outcomes of bimalleolar fractures poorer than those of lateral malleolar fractures with medial ligamentous injury? J Bone Joint Surg Am. 2007;89(7):1438-41.

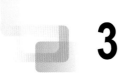

3

Closed Reduction of Shoulder Dislocations

Colin Prensky, Kenneth A Egol

INTRODUCTION

The glenohumeral joint is a ball and socket joint that sacrifices inherent stability for an enhanced range of motion. The shoulder is the most commonly dislocated joint in the body accounting for 50 percent of major joint dislocations seen in the acute setting. Anterior dislocations are by far the most common. However posterior, inferior and multidirectional dislocations are possible. The diagnosis of acute dislocation of the shoulder can be made on the basis of history and physical examination but is often confirmed radiographically, which allows for reliable assessment of direction (Figs 3.1A-C).

Before attempting to reduce the dislocation, it is important to carefully examine the injured shoulder. The axillary nerve and vascular bundle may be injured either as a result of the initial trauma, or as a complication of reduction. It is also important to obtain high quality radiographs. An anteroposterior (AP), Scapular Y and axillary lateral radiographs are needed to confirm the presence and direction of the glenohumeral joint. Bony defects such as fractures and "Hill-Sachs" lesion may also be demonstrated.

There are several techniques for the closed reduction of anterior glenohumeral dislocations. All have relatively high success rates but should be considered based on the availability of analgesia/sedation, the presence of assistants and the ease and time of performing the procedure. Care should be taken to minimize pain and trauma to the patient and forceful reductions should be avoided, if possible,

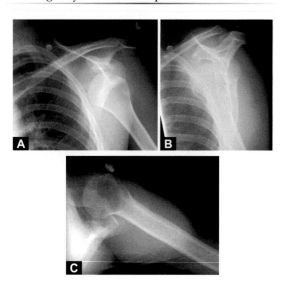

Figs 3.1A-C Anteroposterior, scapular and axillary lateral views of the left shoulder showing evidence of an anterior glenohumeral dislocation

by attempting alternative techniques. For this reason, it is recommended that the clinician to be familiar with several techniques, in case reduction cannot be achieved upon first attempt.

ANTERIOR DISLOCATION

For primary anterior dislocation, prompt reduction will provide the patient with a great deal of pain relief. Reduction may be done with or without anesthesia. Reduction without any anesthesia works best for recurrent or very recent dislocations with limited rotator cuff spasm. Intra-articular lidocaine injection has been shown to be as effective as procedural sedation for the reduction of anterior dislocations while limiting potential drug complications and time spent before discharge. The author suggests the following methods, with more conservative techniques shown first.

■ Scapular Manipulation Technique

In a prone position, the patient hangs the affected arm off the table with 5 to 10 pounds of weight suspended from a strap around the wrist (Fig. 3.2A).

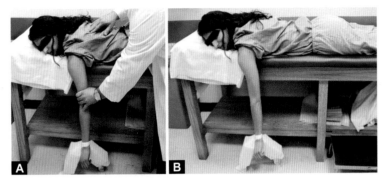

Figs 3.2A and B With the patient in the prone position weights are hung from their wrist on the affected side. The treating practitioner then pushes the inferior tip of the scapula medially while moving the superior aspect laterally facilitating reduction of the glenohumeral joint

The physician uses his or her hands to push the inferior tip of the scapula medially while moving the superior aspect laterally (Fig. 3.2B).

■ External Rotation Technique

This technique is often favored because it may be used to reduce dislocations successfully with little or no analgesia. The technique can be performed with the patient in supine position or seated upright (Fig. 3.3A). If upright, the patient's ipsilateral elbow should be supported to eliminate any traction.

The elbow should be flexed to 90° and the arm is gently externally rotated (Fig. 3.3B). The physician should take care to rotate slowly and pause if the patient experiences pain, in order to allow for muscular relaxation. If the shoulder has not reduced spontaneously by 90° of external rotation, the arm is slowly abducted and the humeral head may be lifted into place.

■ Stimson Technique

This method relies on complete muscle relaxation to be successful. The patient is positioned prone on the gurney or examination table. The injured arm is positioned hanging over the side with 10 to 15 pounds suspended in a similar manner as described above. Reduction should occur within 20 to 30 minutes.

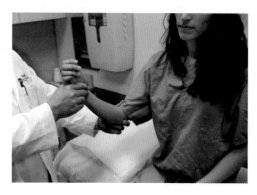

Fig. 3.3A External rotation technique with the patient seated upright

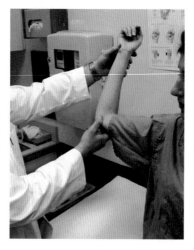

Fig. 3.3B With the elbow flexed to 90 degrees and the shoulder in external rotation the shoulder is slowly brought into abduction facilitating reduction of the glenohumeral joint

■ Milch Technique

With the patient supine, the physician externally rotates and abducts the patient's arm. When the arm reaches the overhead position, the elbow is extended. The physician applies gentle traction. The physician's free hand may be used to manipulate the humeral head over the glenoid labrum.

■ Traction-Countertraction Technique

The patient should be positioned supine, with a sheet tied around the thorax, positioned at the level of the axilla. Using the sheet, an assistant provides countertraction while the physician applies traction to the patient's forearm at an angle of 30° of abduction and forward flexion of 20 to 30° (Figs 3.4A-D). The traction should be gentle and may require a constant application for up to 5 minutes. Sudden forceful movements should be avoided as they may cause additional neurovascular, soft tissue or bony injury to the patient.

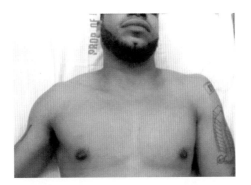

Fig. 3.4A 28-year-old right hand dominant male who presented to the Emergency Room with an acute first time shoulder dislocation. Note the asymmetry present with respect to his shoulder contour

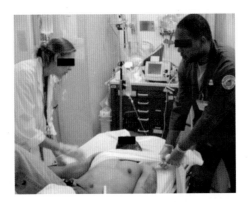

Fig. 3.4B Use of the traction-countertraction technique for glenohumeral reduction

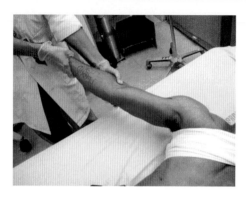

Fig. 3.4C While countertraction is applied, a steady traction force is applied to the affected upper extremity facilitating reduction of the dislocated humeral head

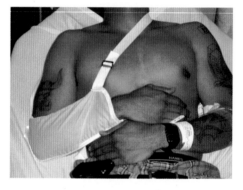

Fig. 3.4D Following successful reduction symmetry is restored and the patient is placed into a sling

■ Modified Hippocratic Technique

The patient should be placed in a supine position with the elbow flexed to 90° and the arm abducted. A sheet is tied and placed around the patient's thorax and an assistant's waist. A second sheet is placed around the patient's proximal forearm and the physician's waist. The physician applies traction to the patient's arm, while countertraction is provided by the assistant. Reduction may require gentle internal and external rotation or manipulation of the proximal humerus.

■ Reduction under Anesthesia

If the above techniques are not successful, reduction under anesthesia may be necessary. This technique may also be required in the setting of significant fracture. Anesthesia allows for complete muscle relaxation and reduction often occurs easily with little risk of additional injury.

POSTERIOR DISLOCATIONS

Posterior glenohumeral dislocations are much less common, accounting for approximately 1 to 2 percent of all glenohumeral dislocations. They are often associated with a history of direct trauma to the anterior shoulder, the strong muscular contractions of epileptic seizures/electric shock, or falls on an outstretched arm. They can be more difficult to detect on physical examination than anterior dislocations, making confirmation with a scapular "Y" radiograph very important. Associated bony lesions include fractures to the posterior glenoid, reversed Hill-Sachs deformity, humeral shaft and lesser tuberosity.

Often, posterior dislocations are accompanied by a high degree of pain and muscular spasm, making analgesia and muscle relaxation extremely important. Reduction technique is applied with the help of an assistant. The patient is positioned supine. The physician applies traction to the humerus with the arm abducted. The assistant gently manipulates the humeral head into the glenoid anteriorly.

INFERIOR DISLOCATIONS

Inferior dislocations, also known as luxatio erecta, are extremely rare. Severe soft tissue trauma and fracture usually accompany inferior dislocation due to the mechanism of injury. A history will usually reveal that the arm was hyperabducted, where the neck of the humerus is forced against the acromion. The acromion acts as a fulcrum, which forces the humeral head down, tearing the inferior capsule.

Physical examination of luxatio erecta is characteristic, with the arm fully abducted. Usually the patient's hand will be resting on or behind his or her head. The humeral head will be easily palpable on the lateral chest.

Reduction is achieved with an assistant through the use of traction and countertraction. The physician applies traction in line with the humerus and the assistant applies countertraction. A noticeable "clunk" demonstrates the reduction.

■ Two-Step Approach

A two-step technique may also be used whereby the luxatio erecta dislocation is converted by the physician to an anterior dislocation after which any of the preferred techniques described above may be used to complete the reduction.

The patient must be placed in a supine position. Sedation may be administered as needed. The physician should stand next to the patient's head on the ipsilateral side to the injury. Facing towards the patient's feet, the physician should place the adjacent hand (superior) on the midshaft of the humerus, while the opposite hand (inferior) is positioned over the medial epicondyle. The inferior hand provides gentle superior force at the distal humerus while the physician uses the superior hand to manipulate the humeral head to the anterior rim of the glenoid from its inferior position. A straight contour of the shoulder and prominence of the posterolateral edge of the acromion demonstrates that the humeral head is now dislocated in an anterior orientation. The physician should be able to adduct the humerus at this point.

At this point, the physician may use whichever anterior dislocation reduction technique that is most comfortable. The authors, Nho et al prefer the external rotation method. They report that the two-step maneuver was successfully completed with a single operator and minimal sedation. They recommend a shoulder trauma series to confirm reduction as well as a careful neurovascular assessment.

POST-REDUCTION CARE

Shoulder immobilization should be recommended for a short period of time following subluxations and dislocations as needed for pain. Studies have not shown a significant effect on post-reduction recurrence based on immobilization time. For primary dislocations, an early range of motion and rotator cuff strengthening program should be recommended; however extreme external rotation or forward flexion should be avoided. A decrease in apprehension to external rotation and abduction is often a good indicator that the patient may return to normal activities if strength has also improved.

Patients younger than 20 years of age are very likely to develop recurrent dislocations due to soft tissue injuries associated with their first dislocation episode. Incidence of recurrent instability is often seen as indirectly proportional to age. Early arthroscopic Bankart repair for primary anterior dislocations has been suggested with positive results in the young, active patient population with patients having fewer recurrences of instability.

SUGGESTED READINGS

1. Acute Anterior Dislocations: Evaluation and Treatment. Arciero R. Chapter 10. In The Unstable Shoulder. Warren, Craig, Altchek ed. 1999. Lippincott-Raven. Philadelphia, PA

2. Position and duration of immobilization after primary anterior shoulder dislocation: a systematic review and meta-analysis of the literature. Paterson WH, Throckmorton TW, Koester M, Azar FM, Kuhn JE. J Bone Joint Surg Am. 2010 Dec 15;92(18):2924-33. Review.

3. Management of acute glenohumeral dislocations. Sileo MJ, Joseph S, Nelson CO, Botts JD, Penna J. Am J Orthop (Belle Mead NJ). 2009 Jun;38(6):282-90. Review

4. Treating the initial anterior shoulder dislocation--an evidence-based medicine approach. Kuhn JE. Sports Med Arthrosc. 2006 Dec;14(4):192-8. Review.

5. Anterior shoulder dislocation: a review of reduction techniques. Riebel GD, McCabe JB. Am J Emerg Med. 1991 Mar;9(2):180-8. Review. No abstract available.

6. Posterior shoulder dislocations and fracture-dislocations. Robinson CM, Aderinto J. J Bone Joint Surg Am. 2005 Mar;87(3):639-50. Review.

7. The two-step maneuver for closed reduction of inferior glenohumeral dislocation (luxatio erecta to anterior dislocation to reduction). Nho SJ, Dodson CC, Bardzik KF, Brophy RH, Domb BG, MacGillivray JD. J Orthop Trauma. 2006 May;20(5):354-7.

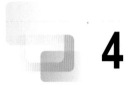

4

Closed Reduction of Elbow Dislocations

Sonya Khurana, Eric J Strauss

INTRODUCTION

Elbow dislocations are fairly common injuries accounting for 20 percent of all traumatic dislocations. The elbow most commonly dislocates in the posterior or posterolateral direction. Posterior elbow dislocations are the most common dislocations in children less than ten years of age. Elbow dislocations most commonly occur after a twisting injury or fall onto an outstretched arm and result in a ruptured capsule.

ANATOMY OF THE ELBOW

The elbow joint has three articulations between the radius, ulna and the humerus. The medial collateral ligament resists valgus force and the lateral collateral ligament prevents rotational instability between the distal humerus and proximal radius and ulna. The medial collateral ligament is composed of anterior and posterior portions. The anterior portion runs from the medial epicondyle of the humerus to the medial margin of the coronoid process (sublime tubercle). The posterior portion runs from the distal and posterior aspect of the medial epicondyle of the femur to the medial margin of the olecranon. The ulnar band of the lateral collateral ligament runs from a depression below the lateral epicondyle of the humerus to the ulna (crista supinatoris). The annular ligament circles the radial head and keeps the radius in contact with the radial notch of the ulna.

The ulnar nerve passes posterior and medial to the elbow joint through the cubital tunnel, which extends from the medial epidcondyle to the olecranon. The roof of the tunnel (Osborne's ligament) is an aponeurosis and the floor is made up of the medial collateral ligament, joint capsule and olecranon. The radial nerve originates from the posterior cord of the brachial plexus and passes anterior to the lateral epicondyle when it reaches the distal part of the humerus.

The cubital fossa contains the radial nerve, median nerve and brachial artery. It is bounded by the distance between the medial and lateral epicondyles of the humerus superiorly; medially by the lateral border of the pronator teres and laterally by the medial border of the brachioradialis.

EMERGENCY ROOM EVALUATION

When taking the history of the patient with a suspected elbow dislocation, it is important to note the mechanism of injury, the type and location of pain, the presence of any sensory, motor or vascular deficits, the time of injury, and whether or not the patient has a history of a prior elbow injury. When performing the physical examination, it is important to note the presence of gross deformity and the condition of the overlying soft tissue. The elbow should be evaluated for the presence of an effusion, put through a range of motion and undergo stability testing if possible. These findings should be compared to the uninjured contralateral side.

In an uninjured elbow, the medial and lateral epicondyles form an isosceles triangle with the olecranon. This anatomical triangle will not be present if the patient has a simple elbow dislocation (no fracture present) as the relationship between the olecranon and the epicondyles will be altered, and the olecranon process will become more prominent. There may also be an empty area medially. The triangle will be maintained in the setting of a supracondylar fracture rather than an elbow dislocation.

Neurovascular injury is uncommon but a thorough evaluation is warranted and the evaluator should be alert for the development of compartment syndrome. Up to 10 percent of patients will develop an ulnar nerve neuropathy with decreased sensation in the medial one and half digits starting from the wrist and extending up to the tips of the digits and/or difficulty in abducting the digits. Median nerve injury is rare and is characterized by severe pain that does not improve with the reduction. The patient will have difficulty in abducting the thumb and/or loss of sensation of the palmar aspect of the skin from the wrist to the tips of the lateral three and a half digits and dorsal aspect of the distal two-third of these same digits. Brachial artery injury is also rare and is characterized by radiating pain, decreased skin temperature and pallor in the distal arm. Due to rich collateral circulation about the elbow, distal pulses do not preclude a more proximal arterial injury. Posterior interosseous nerve (a branch of the radial nerve) injury is characterized by loss of sensation on the dorsal aspect of the hand, from the wrist to the proximal one-third of the lateral 3.5 digits.

RADIOGRAPHIC EVALUATION

In addition to documenting the direction of the elbow dislocation, proper radiographic views are important to rule out the presence of concomitant fractures of the distal humerus, olecranon or radial head. It is important to obtain a true lateral view of the elbow (Fig. 4.1), an anteroposterior view of the forearm and the humerus.

REDUCTION AND IMMOBILIZATION OF A SIMPLE ELBOW DISLOCATION

After ruling out any associated elbow fractures, reduction, as outlined below, is necessary. Following successful reduction, the patient will be placed in a posterior elbow splint with a side bar with the elbow in approximately 90° of flexion.

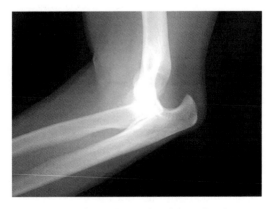

Fig. 4.1 Lateral view of the elbow showing a simple posterolateral dislocation of the elbow

■ Steps for Reduction

- Ensure the patient has an adequate pain control. This may be done with an intra-articular anesthetic and/or pain medications. If these measures are ineffective, the patient may be put under conscious sedation.
- Remove clothing and jewelry from the affected limb.
- Place the patient in the supine position.
- Align the olecranon and distal humerus in the medial-lateral plane (Fig. 4.2).
- Supinate the forearm.
- Apply upward traction across elbow while flexing the elbow to 90° (Fig. 4.3).
- Have assistant apply countertraction and stabilize the humeral shaft.
- Place thumb on top of the patient's olecranon process and lever the olecranon over the distal humerus with direct pressure. The force from the thumb should be directed upward and posterior while the arm is flexed up to 90°. A palpable "clunk" should be felt.
- Check stability by taking the elbow through a complete arc of motion.
- Confirm successful reduction by checking for smooth and unrestricted arc of motion and realignment of the olecranon, medial and lateral epicondyles into the isosceles triangle.

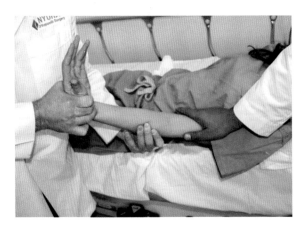

Fig. 4.2 With the patient in the supine position, the treating practitioner aligns the olecranon and distal humerus

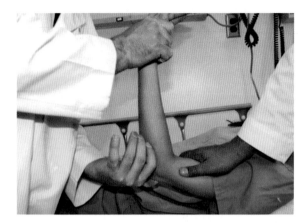

Fig. 4.3 Reduction maneuver with the application of traction across the elbow. Note the treating practitioner's left thumb pushing on the olecranon tip facilitating reduction of the ulnohumeral articulation

- After confirming a stable and successful reduction, apply a padded posterior splint to immobilize the elbow in approximately 90° flexion and forearm in neutral rotation (please refer to the following section for instructions on how to apply a posterior splint). Post-reduction radiographs must confirm concentric ulnohumeral and radiocapitellar reductions (Figs 4.4A and B).

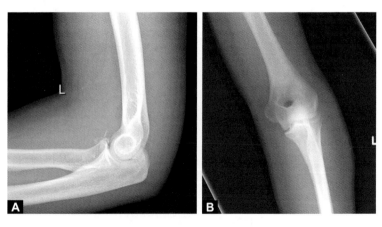

Figs 4.4A and B Post-reduction lateral and anteroposterior views of the left elbow confirming concentric ulnohumeral and radiocapitellar reductions. On the lateral view note the presence of a small coronoid fracture associated with the dislocation event

The splint can be discarded within 1 to 2 weeks. Make sure the splint extends far enough to support the wrist and keep the elbow above the heart to help reduce swelling.

- Patient should be re-evaluated by an orthopedic surgeon 7 to 10 days following the injury for re-evaluation of elbow stability and referral for physical therapy.

■ Applications of Posterior Long Arm Splint

Materials

Materials required are plaster rolls of 8 to 10 sheets of 3 or 4 inches, depending on the patient's size, 1 inch plaster roll, cotton undercast padding, a basin of lukewarm water, elastic bandages 3 to 4 inches wide, chux pads, trauma shears, bedsheet and stockinette as shown in Figure 4.5.

- Make sure the patient is comfortably positioned.
- Remove clothing and jewellery from the affected limb.
- Cover the patient with a sheet to protect him/her from splatter from the plaster.
- Flex the affected elbow to 90°, extend the wrist to 10 to 20° and keep the forearm in neutral position with the thumb up.
- Wrap the arm in cotton padding, starting distally and moving proximally, and overlapping each layer by half a width (Fig. 4.6). The cotton padding should extend 2 to 3 cm beyond the plaster.

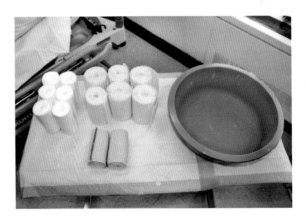

Fig. 4.5 Materials required for splinting

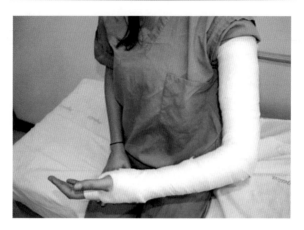

Fig. 4.6 With the elbow in approximately 80–90° of flexion and the wrist in 10–20° of extension, wrap the affected arm in cotton undercast padding

Smooth out creases and wrinkles, as these can cause pressure and damage underlying soft tissue. Make sure to add extra padding to bony prominences of the elbow and wrist, epicondyles of the elbow, metacarpophalangeal joints and the base of the thumb. Remove excessive padding from cubital fossa.

- Measure the plaster by placing one end of a dry roll of plaster on the ulnar side of the affected arm, extending from the palmar crease to the proximal humerus. Add about 5 mm of extra plaster on either end, as plaster shrinks when it is wet. Pinch off this desired length and fold over the plaster. Unroll the rest of the plaster and fold over until there are total 8 to 10 layers (Figs 4.7A and B). A supporting side slab is also measured out.
- Immerse the plaster in the room temperature water and squeeze out the excess water. Lay the plaster flat and smooth out the wrinkles and folds.
- Apply the wet plaster over the padding, starting on the ulnar side at the mid-metacarpals and continuing to the proximal humerus (Fig. 4.8). Have the patient use the opposite hand to hold the distal end of the wet plaster. If the patient cannot do it, an assistant must be called in to do so.
- Smooth out the excess plaster at the elbow and mold it against the outside splint.
- Reinforce the splint with the supporting side slab extending from the mid-humerus to mid-forearm (Fig. 4.9).

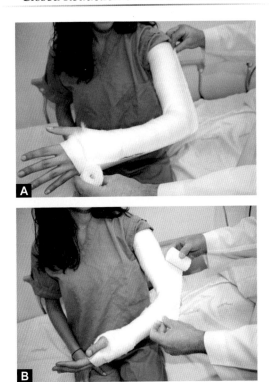

Figs 4.7A and B The appropriate lengths of the posterior component and lateral supporting slab are measured out

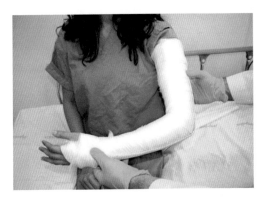

Fig. 4.8 The rolled out posterior component of the splint is dipped in luke-warm water and applied to the posterior aspect of the affected upper extremity

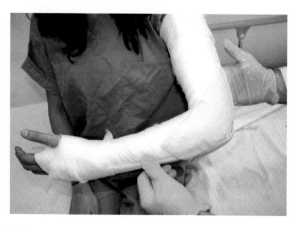

Fig. 4.9 The supporting side slab is then applied extending from the mid-humerus level to the mid-forearm level

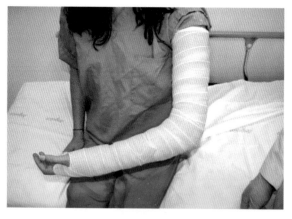

Fig. 4.10 The splint is then overwrapped with an ACE bandage

- Apply the elastic wrap over the wet plaster, starting distally and moving proximally (Fig. 4.10). Do not wrap too tightly and ensure an adequate hole for the thumb.
- Mold the splint into the desired shape while the plaster is still wet and tell the patient to keep his or her hand, forearm, wrist and elbow immobile until the plaster dries.

- Inform the patient that he or she may feel some warmth as the splint dries. However, if the heat becomes too intense, remove the splint as thermal burns can occur.
- Check neurovascular function after the splint dries.

SUGGESTED READINGS

1. Carter Sadie J, Carl A Germann, Angelo A Dacus, et al. "Orthopedic pitfalls in the ED: neurovascular injury associated with posterior elbow dislocations." Am J Emerg Med. 2010;28(8):960-5. Epub 2010 Mar 12.
2. De Haan J, Schep NW, Tuinebreijer WE, et al. Simple elbow dislocations: a systematic review of the literature. Arch Orthop Trauma Surg. 2010;130(2):241-9. Epub 2009 Apr 2.
3. Joseph Chorley. (2009, July 13). Elbow injuries in the young athlete [online]. Available from http://www.uptodate.com/online/content/topic.do?topicKey=ped_trau/13894&selectedTitle=1%7E150&source=search_result
4. Maripuri SN, Debnath UK, Rao P, et al. Simple elbow dislocation among adults: a comparative study of two different methods of treatment. Injury. 2007;38(11):1254-8. Epub 2007 Jul 20.
5. McCullough L. Splinting, posterior elbow: treatment and medication [online]. Available from http://emedicine.medscape.com/article/80089-treatment
6. Swiontkowski MF, Stovitz SD. Manual of Orthopaedics. Philadelphia, PA: Lippincott Williams & Wilkins; 2006.
7. Wheeless CR. (2009, September 26). Anterior interosseous branch of median nerve [online]. Available from http://www.wheelessonline.com/ortho/anterior_interosseous_branch_of_median_nerve
8. Yallapragada RK, Patko JT. Elbow collateral ligaments [online]. Available from http://emedicine.medscape.com/article/1230902-overview

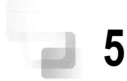

5

Joint Aspiration and Injection Techniques

Eric J Strauss

INTRODUCTION

Joint space aspirations and intra-articular injections are common procedures performed for both diagnostic and therapeutic purposes. Synovial fluid obtained from a successful joint aspiration can be used to rule out the presence of infection, identify a crystalline arthropathy or relieve pain from symptomatic effusion or hemarthrosis. For a variety of conditions, intra-articular administration of medications, such as corticosteroids and hyaluronic acid, can provide patients with significant benefits including pain relief and functional improvement. Knowledge of techniques for accurate and reproducible joint aspirations and injections are essential skills for the practicing healthcare practitioners and require a thorough understanding of both the relevant anatomy and aseptic protocols. Common sites for aspiration and injection procedures include the shoulder, elbow, wrist, knee and ankle joints.

NECESSARY MATERIALS

Various necessary materials required for joint aspirations are described as follows and shown in Figure 5.1.

- Sterile gloves
- Syringes (size depends on anticipated amount of fluid to be aspirated or the volume of medication to be injected; knee and

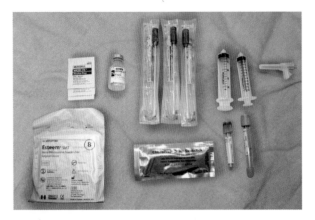

Fig. 5.1 Necessary supplies and materials for joint aspiration and intra-articular injection

shoulder injections are typically performed using 10 cc syringes, elbow and ankle injections are typically performed using 5 cc syringes).

- Needles [size depends on the indication; joint injections are usually performed with a 22-or 25-gauge needle, aspirations may require larger bore needles (18-20-gauge) especially if a hemarthrosis is being aspirated].
- Povidone-iodine solution is required for skin prep.
- Culture sticks (aerobic and anaerobic) and a purple top tube (for cell count) if the aspiration is being performed to rule out septic arthritis.
- Yellow top or red speckle top tube if the aspiration is being performed to diagnose a crystalline arthropathy.
- Prepared corticosteroid-lidocaine (1cc:9cc ratio for knee and shoulder injections, 1cc:4cc ratio for ankle and elbow injections) syringe for injection or hyaluronic acid syringe.
- Ethyl chloride spray (a topical analgesic) may be utilized.
- Hemostat (can be used to facilitate disconnection of the needle from the syringe if additional syringes are needed).
- Alcohol swabs.
- Gauze pads.
- Band-aid.

SHOULDER ASPIRATION AND INJECTION TECHNIQUE

The glenohumeral joint is often aspirated as a part of the work up in ruling out septic or inflammatory arthritis and injected with corticosteroids and/or lidocaine as a part of the treatment of adhesive capsulitis, symptomatic SLAP tears and glenohumeral arthritis. Patients with symptoms and functional limitations secondary to rotator cuff tendinopathy, long head of the biceps tendonitis and subdeltoid bursitis unresponsive to oral anti-inflammatory medications and physical therapy are often indicated for subacromial space injections. A number of approaches to the aspiration and injection of the shoulder have been described, with the anterior and posterior approaches most commonly used.

▋ Posterior Approach for Both Glenohumeral and Subacromial Aspirations/Injections

- Patient is placed in the seated position with their affected upper extremity resting comfortably at their side on the chair's arm rest with the shoulder in an internally rotated position.
- Examine the posterolateral aspect of the shoulder looking for evidence of overlying cellulitis (avoid placing the needle through any area of potential infection).
- Palpate the posterior and lateral borders of the acromion process localizing its most posterolateral aspect and palpate the coracoid process anteriorly.
- Localize the posterolateral soft spot between the humeral head and the glenoid approximately two fingerbreadths distal and one fingerbreadth medial to the posterolateral corner of the acromion (The location of the humeral head relative to the glenoid can be appreciated with rotation of the upper arm). Mark this site as the starting point for the aspiration/injection (Fig. 5.2). The same starting point has been used for both glenohumeral injection and subacromial injection.
- Prep the skin in this region using alcohol and povidone-iodine.
- Put on sterile gloves.
- For aspiration, use a 18-20-gauge needle attached to the appropriately sized syringe (typically a 10–20 cc syringe will be used).

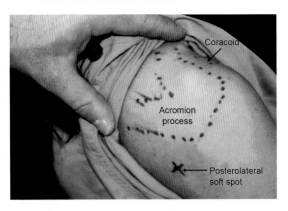

Fig. 5.2 Both subacromial and intra-articular glenohumeral injections are given via the posterolateral portal site which is located two fingerbreadths distal and one fingerbreadth medial to the posterolateral aspect of the acromion process

- If available, an assistant can spray the area with ethyl chloride spray to provide superficial analgesia just prior to needle insertion.
- The needle should be directed anteriorly toward the coracoid process advancing slowly aiming slightly medial (Fig. 5.3). Any contact with underlying bone of the humeral head should prompt a careful retraction and redirection of the needle more medially and slightly more superiorly.

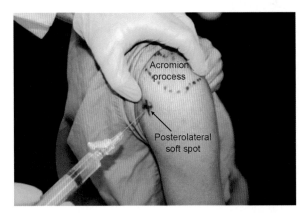

Fig. 5.3 The needle is inserted aiming toward the coracoid process

- Once the needle is injected in the intra-articular space, start aspirating.
- If necessary, additional syringes can be used for aspiration by disconnecting the luer lock from the needle. One can use a hemostat to stabilize the needle taking care to avoid changing its intra-articular position.
- Once the aspiration is complete, a new sterile needle can be attached to the syringe allowing for distribution of the obtained fluid into culture tubes and blood tubes for later analysis (assistant can be helpful during this step to ensure maintenance of sterility).
- For injections, the same approach can be used injecting the prepared medication once the needle is within the intra-articular space.
- When injecting medication into the subacromial space, the same starting point is used with the needle aimed superiorly at a 10 to 15° angle to end up just distal to the undersurface of the acromion process.
- Once in the subacromial space, aspirate first to ensure that the tip of the needle is not intravascular followed by injection of the prepared lidocaine-corticosteroid mixture.
- Following the aspiration and/or injection the needle is removed from the knee. The prepped skin is cleaned with an alcohol swab, dried with a gauze pad and a band-aid is applied.

Anterior Approach for Glenohumeral Aspirations/Injections

- Patient is placed in the seated position with their affected upper extremity resting comfortably at their side on the chair's arm rest with the shoulder in a neutral or slightly externally rotated (approximately 15 to 20°) position.
- Examine the anterior aspect of the shoulder looking for evidence of overlying cellulitis (avoid placing the needle through any area of potential infection).
- Palpate the coracoid process and the humeral head (rotation of the upper extremity can help localize the humeral head relative to the glenoid).
- Mark the starting point for the aspiration/injection just medial to the humeral head, 5 to 10 mm lateral to the tip of the coracoid process (Fig. 5.4).

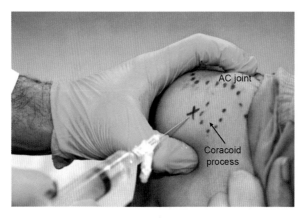

Fig. 5.4 Marking the starting point for glenohumeral injections (anterior approach)

- Prepare the skin in this region using alcohol and povidone-iodine.
- Put on sterile gloves.
- For aspiration, use a 20- or 21-gauge needle attached to the appropriately sized syringe (typically a 10–20 cc syringe will be used).
- If available, an assistant can spray the area with ethyl chloride spray to provide superficial analgesia just prior to needle insertion.
- The needle should be directed posteriorly aiming slightly lateral and slightly superior in an effort to penetrate the joint in the region of the rotator interval. Any contact with underlying bone of the humeral head should prompt a careful retraction and redirection of the needle more medially and slightly more superiorly, contact with the bone of the glenoid should prompt redirection further laterally.
- Once in the intra-articular space, start aspirating.
- If necessary, additional syringes can be used for aspiration by disconnecting the luer lock from the needle. One can use a hemostat to stabilize the needle taking care to avoid changing its intra-articular position.
- Once the aspiration is complete, a new sterile needle can be attached to the syringe allowing for distribution of the obtained fluid into culture tubes and blood tubes for later analysis (assistant can be helpful during this step to ensure maintenance of sterility).

- For injections, the same approach can be used injecting the prepared medication once the needle is within the intra-articular space.
- When injecting medication into the subacromial space, the same starting point is used with the needle aimed superiorly at a 10 to 15° angle to end up just distal to the undersurface of the acromion process.

ELBOW ASPIRATION AND INJECTION TECHNIQUE

Access to the elbow joint can be reproducibly achieved via a lateral approach understanding the local anatomy and relationship between the olecranon process, the lateral epicondyle of the humerus and the radial head. Elbow aspirations and injections can be very useful in the setting of symptomatic effusions from arthritis (inflammatory and osteoarthritis) and in the diagnosis and management of radial head fractures. In the setting of elbow trauma, intra-articular aspiration can help identify an occult fracture (if blood with or without fat globules is identified) in addition of providing pain relief and improved range of motion following injection of local anesthetic into the joint space.

■ Steps

- Patient is placed in the supine position on the examination table with the affected elbow at 45° of flexion and the hand in neutral position.
- Examine the lateral aspect of the elbow looking for evidence of overlying cellulitis (avoid placing the needle through any area of potential infection).
- Palpate and mark out the tip of the olecranon process posteriorly, the lateral epicondyle proximally and the radial head distally. Rotation of the patient's forearm may facilitate accurate localization of the radial head. These three bony landmarks create a triangle within which a "soft spot" can be palpated and marked out as the starting point for the aspiration/injection (Fig. 5.5).
- Prep the skin in this region using alcohol and povidone-iodine.
- Put on sterile gloves.
- For aspiration, use a 20- or 21-gauge needle attached to the appropriately sized syringe (typically a 5 cc syringe will be used).

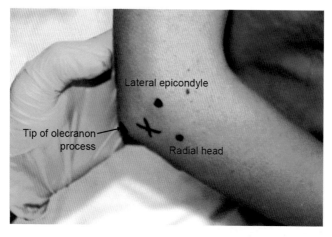

Fig. 5.5 Marking the starting point for elbow aspirations and injections

- If available, an assistant can spray the area with ethyl chloride spray to provide superficial analgesia just prior to needle insertion.
- The needle should be directed toward the medial epicondyle, advancing slowly aiming slightly posterior and slightly distal (Fig. 5.6). Any contact with the underlying bone should prompt a careful retraction and redirection of the needle.
- Once the needle is injected in the intra-articular space, start aspirating.
- If necessary, additional syringes can be used for aspiration by disconnecting the luer lock from the needle. One can use a hemostat to stabilize the needle taking care to avoid changing its intra-articular position.
- Once the aspiration is complete, a new sterile needle can be attached to the syringe allowing for distribution of the obtained fluid into culture tubes and blood tubes for later analysis (assistant can be helpful during this step to ensure maintenance of sterility).
- For injections, the same approach is used injecting the prepared medication once the needle is within the intra-articular space.
- Following the aspiration and/or injection, the needle is removed from the knee. The prepped skin is cleaned with an alcohol swab, dried with a gauze pad and a band-aid is applied.

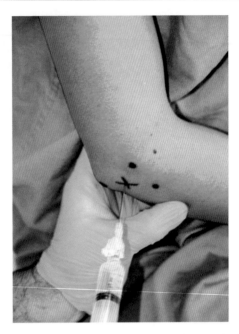

Fig. 5.6 For aspiration/injection of the elbow the needle is directed toward the medial epicondyle

WRIST ASPIRATION AND INJECTION TECHNIQUE

The safest and most reproducible access to the wrist joint is from a dorsal approach. Since most of the intercarpal joint spaces communicate with the radiocarpal articulation, the dorsal technique for aspiration and injection is the most commonly used in the diagnosis of septic arthritis or crystalline arthropathy, removal of painful effusions and the administration of intra-articular medications.

■ Steps

- Patient can be placed either in the supine position or in a comfortable recumbent position. In the supine position, the wrist can be placed on the patient's abdomen utilizing a folded sheet or gown to place the wrist in a slightly palmar-flexed position which will facilitate access to the radiocarpal joint.
- Examine the dorsal aspect of the wrist looking for evidence of overlying cellulitis (avoid placing the needle through any area of potential infection).

- Palpate the distal aspect of the distal radius and the borders of the anatomic snuff box. A soft spot can usually be palpated ulnar to the extensor pollicis longus and extensor carpi radialis brevis just distal to the end of the distal radius. Mark this spot using a pen or marker (Fig. 5.7).
- Prep the skin in this region using alcohol and povidone-iodine.
- Put on sterile gloves.
- For aspiration, use a 20- or 21-gauge needle attached to the appropriately sized syringe (typically a 5 cc syringe will be used).
- If available, an assistant can spray the area with ethyl chloride spray to provide superficial analgesia just prior to needle insertion.
- The needle should be directed perpendicular to the skin directed slightly distal and slightly radial into the intra-articular space (Fig. 5.8). If the needle tip hits the bone of the distal radius, gently pull it back and redirect it distally and slightly more radial (toward the thumb).
- Once within the intra-articular space, start aspirating.
- If necessary, additional syringes can be used for aspiration by disconnecting the luer lock from the needle. One can use a

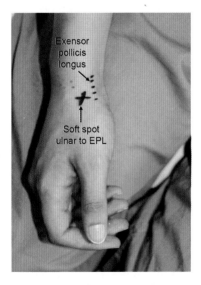

Fig. 5.7 The starting point for wrist aspiration/injection can be found as a soft spot ulnar to the extensor pollicis longus (EPL) tendon

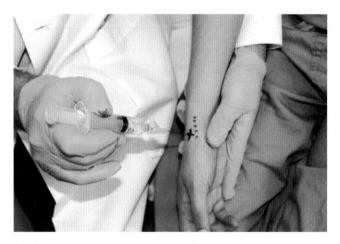

Fig. 5.8 The needle is inserted into the intra-articular space of the wrist between the scaphoid and distal radius

hemostat to stabilize the needle taking care to avoid changing its intra-articular position.

- Once the aspiration is complete, a new sterile needle can be attached to the syringe allowing for distribution of the obtained fluid into culture tubes and blood tubes for later analysis (assistant can be helpful during this step to ensure maintenance of sterility).
- For injections, the same approach can be used injecting the prepared medication once the needle is within the intra-articular space.
- Following the aspiration and/or injection, the needle is removed from the knee. The prepped skin is cleaned with an alcohol swab, dried with a gauze pad and a band-aid is applied.

KNEE ASPIRATION AND INJECTION TECHNIQUE

The knee joint is the most commonly aspirated and injected joint in the body. Knee aspirations and injections are used to establish diagnoses, relieve pain by removing hematomas or synovial fluid and for the instillation of various medications. A variety of approaches have been described for access to the intra-articular space of the knee (superolateral, superomedial, inferolateral and inferomedial). The superolateral aspiration and injection has been shown to be the most accurate and reproducible (93% accuracy as compared to 71–75% for the inferomedial and inferolateral approaches).

■ Superolateral Approach

- Patient in the supine position with the knee fully extended.
- Examine the knee to determine the approximate amount of joint fluid present (will dictate the size of syringe utilized for aspiration) and look for evidence of overlying cellulitis (avoid placing the needle through any area of potential infection).
- Palpate the superolateral aspect of the patella and mark the skin one fingerbreadth superior and one fingerbreadth lateral to this location as the starting point (Fig. 5.9).
- Prep the skin in this region using alcohol and povidone-iodine.
- Put on sterile gloves.
- For aspiration, use an 18-20-gauge needle attached to the appropriately sized syringe.
- The non-dominant hand can be used to evert the patella slightly, increasing the available space and ease of needle insertion into the intra-articular space.
- If available, an assistant can spray the area with ethyl chloride spray to provide superficial analgesia just prior to needle insertion.

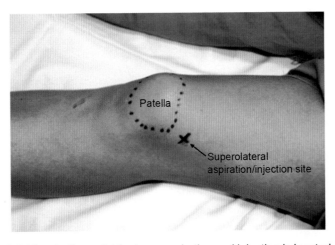

Fig. 5.9 The starting point for knee aspiration and injection is located one fingerbreadth superior and one fingerbreadth lateral to the superolateral aspect of the patella

- The needle should be directed 45° distally and 45° posteriorly into the intra-articular space with care taken to avoid hitting the articular surfaces of the patella or corresponding trochlea (Fig. 5.10).
- Once in the intra-articular space, begin aspirating. One can facilitate synovial fluid egress by using the non-dominant hand to compress the opposite side of the knee.
- If necessary, additional syringes can be used for aspiration by disconnecting the luer lock from the needle. One can use a hemostat to stabilize the needle taking care to avoid changing its intra-articular position.
- Once the aspiration is complete, a new sterile needle can be attached to the syringe allowing for distribution of the obtained fluid into culture tubes and blood tubes for later analysis (assistant can be helpful during this step to ensure maintenance of sterility).
- For injections, the same approach can be used injecting the prepared medication once the needle is within the intra-articular space.
- Following the aspiration and/or injection the needle is removed from the knee. The prepped skin is cleaned with an alcohol swab, dried with a gauze pad and a band-aid is applied.

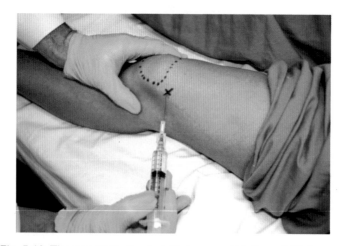

Fig. 5.10 The needle is directed 45 degrees distally and 45 degrees posteriorly into the intra-articular space

■ Inferolateral Approach

- Place the patient in the seated position with the knee flexed over the end of the examination table to 90°.
- Palpate the inferior pole of the patella. The lateral aspect of the patellar tendon and the proximal aspect of the lateral tibial plateau. A palpable "soft spot" should be present one finger-breadth proximal to the lateral tibial plateau just lateral to the lateral aspect of the patellar tendon. Mark this location as the starting point for the aspiration/injection (Fig. 5.11).
- Prep the skin in this region using alcohol and povidone-iodine.
- Put on sterile gloves.
- For aspiration, use a 20- or 21-gauge needle attached to the appropriately sized syringe.
- If available, an assistant can spray the area with ethyl chloride spray to provide superficial analgesia just prior to needle insertion.
- The needle should be directed from the soft spot starting point approximately 30° medially toward the intercondylar notch taking care to avoid contacting the articular surface of the femoral condyle (Fig. 5.12).

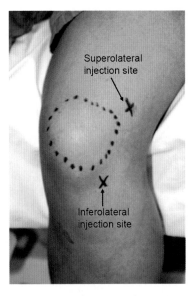

Fig. 5.11 Marking the starting point for aspiration/injection
(inferolateral approach)

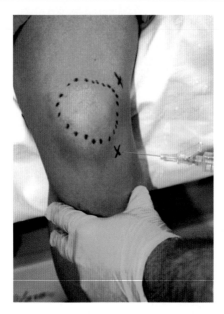

Fig. 5.12 The needle is inserted aiming medially toward the intercondylar notch

- Once in the intra-articular space start aspirating, one can facilitate synovial fluid egress by using the nondominant hand to compress the superior aspect of the knee starting in the suprapatellar region.
- If necessary, additional syringes can be used for aspiration by disconnecting the luer lock from the needle. One can use a hemostat to stabilize the needle taking care to avoid changing its intra-articular position.
- Once the aspiration is complete, a new sterile needle can be attached to the syringe allowing for distribution of the obtained fluid into culture tubes and blood tubes for later analysis.
- For injections, the same approach can be used injecting the prepared medication once the needle is within the intra-articular space.
- Following the aspiration and/or injection the needle is removed from the knee. The prepped skin is cleaned with an alcohol swab, dried with a gauze pad and a band-aid is applied.

ANKLE ASPIRATION AND INJECTION TECHNIQUE

Similar to the other commonly injected joints, aspiration and injection of the ankle joint is indicated for identification of infection and crystal deposition disease in addition to providing corticosteroids to treat symptoms associated with inflammation. An anteromedial approach is typically utilized as it provides consistent access to the ankle joint while avoiding injury to the superficial peroneal nerve.

◼ Steps

- Patient in the supine position with the ankle in a relaxed position. A bump is placed posterior to the distal tibia to help facilitate proper positioning.
- Palpate the anatomy of the ankle noting the anteromedial border of the medial malleolus and the course of the tibialis anterior tendon. Resisted ankle dorsiflexion can help accurately identify the tibialis anterior tendon.
- Mark the space between the medial malleolus and the tibialis anterior tendon feeling for the articulation between the tibial plafond and the dome of the talus (Fig. 5.13).
- Prepare the skin in this region using alcohol and povidone-iodine.
- Put on sterile gloves.
- For aspiration, use an 18-20-gauge needle attached to the appropriately sized syringe.
- If available, an assistant can spray the area with ethyl chloride spray to provide superficial analgesia just prior to needle insertion.
- The needle should be directed posterolaterally, slowly advancing to avoid injury to the articular surfaces of the talus or the distal tibia (Fig. 5.14).
- Once in the intra-articular space start aspirating.
- Once the aspiration is complete, a new sterile needle can be attached to the syringe allowing for distribution of the obtained fluid into culture tubes and blood tubes for later analysis (assistant can be helpful during this step to ensure maintenance of sterility).
- For injections, the same approach may be used injecting the prepared medication once the needle is within the intra-articular space.

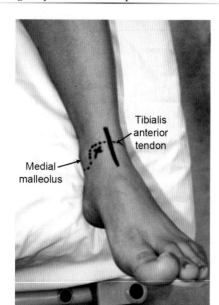

Fig. 5.13 The intra-articular space of the ankle is accessed through a space located between the medial malleolus and the tibialis anterior tendon

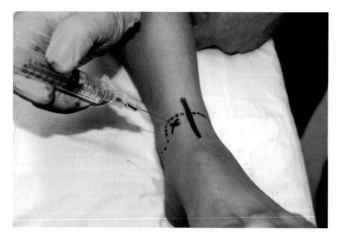

Fig. 5.14 The needle is directed posterolaterally into the intra-articular space

- Following the aspiration and/or injection the needle is removed from the knee. The prepped skin is cleaned with an alcohol swab, dried with a gauze pad and a band-aid is applied.

SUGGESTED READINGS

1. Cardone DA, Tallia AF. Diagnostic and therapeutic injection of the hip and knee. Am Fam Physician. 2003;67(10):2147-52. Review.
2. Cardone DA, Tallia AF. Joint and soft tissue injection. Am Fam Physician. 2002 Jul 15;66(2):283-8.
3. Courtney P, Doherty M. Joint aspiration and injection and synovial fluid analysis. Best Pract Res Clin Rheumatol. 2009;23(2):161-92. Review
4. Pascual E, Doherty M. Aspiration of normal or asymptomatic pathological joints for diagnosis and research: indications, technique and success rate. Ann Rheum Dis. 2009;68(1):3-7. Epub 2008 Apr 2. Review.
5. Patel RV, Haddad FS. Technique of knee joint aspiration. Br J Hosp Med (Lond). 2007;68(6):M100-1. Review. No abstract available.
6. Rifat SF, Moeller JL. Injection and aspiration techniques for the primary care physician. Compr Ther. 2002 Winter;28(4):222-9. Review.
7. Tallia AF, Cardone DA. Diagnostic and therapeutic injection of the ankle and foot. Am Fam Physician. 2003;68(7):1356-62. Review.
8. Tallia AF, Cardone DA. Diagnostic and therapeutic injection of the wrist and hand region. Am Fam Physician. 2003 Feb 15;67(4):745-50. Review

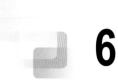

6

Reduction of the Dislocated Total Hip Arthroplasty

Colin Prenksy, Kenneth A Egol

INTRODUCTION

Dislocation is a feared complication following total hip arthroplasty (THA) that leads to pain, functional impairment and serious patient distress. The incidence is reported as high as 7 percent following THA and up to 25 percent after revision arthroplasty. Dislocations occurring within three months of surgery are defined as early dislocations and carry a better prognosis than late dislocations. Due to it multifactorial etiology, including chronic soft tissue laxity and prosthetic wear, late dislocations have a higher rate of recurrent instability.

Risk factors for hip dislocation following THA can be divided into patient risk factors and surgical risk factors derived from the initial arthroplasty. Patient risk factors include a history of alcohol abuse, old age, cognitive impairment/dementia, neuromuscular impairment or muscular weakness, inflammatory arthropathies and a history of osteonecrosis. Inability to adhere properly to post-surgical protocol is also a major factor in early dislocations. Previously, female gender was reported as a risk factor, however recent studies have failed to substantiate this. Certain technical factors related to the index arthroplasty procedure such as the operative approach utilized and component malposition have been shown to increase risk for dislocation. Some studies have demonstrated increased dislocation rates in patients in whom a posterior operative approach was used, malposition of components and inadequate soft tissue tension resulting in laxity. The acetabular component must be positioned to allow safe range of motion without impingement. A cup in 30° of abduction and 20 to 40° anteversion is standard. The design of components and excessive component wear also contribute to the potential for joint instability. Well-positioned components may still dislocate due to impingement on osteophytes and/or soft tissues that are not fully recognized at the time of surgery.

CLINICAL EVALUATION

The patient's history can provide clues to the direction of dislocation. Typically, an anterior dislocation is the result of excessive extension, adduction and external rotation. Conversely, a posterior dislocation usually results from flexion, adduction and internal rotation The history should also include surgical notes, if possible, to understand perioperative joint stability.

While most native hip dislocations result from high energy trauma such as motor vehicle accidents, dislocations of the THA are usually the result of low energy trauma. A patient history should provide information regarding the mechanism of injury. Often the patient will report feeling a distinct "clunking" sensation directly followed by intense hip, thigh and groin pain. The patient will also report extreme difficulty with ambulation and limited range of motion. If the patient's mechanism of injury is high energy, it is also important to perform a full-body trauma assessment. Access to the patient's surgical notes is also helpful during the assessment when evaluating any potential surgical factors.

The physical exam should include both lower extremities. Visual assessment should evaluate the injured limb for shortening and/or malrotation. Comparing the contralateral side for symmetry is helpful. There are several visual clues to direction of dislocation.

The femoral head may be palpated in its dislocated position. A large hematoma may be present. Due to the possibility of neurovascular injury caused by the dislocation as well as reduction, it is extremely important to fully examine the lower extremities and document neurovascular status.

Fluoroscopy can be useful in evaluating the direction of displacement, the position of components and whether the components are stable. Loosening of either the femoral or acetabular component likely will require surgical intervention. Radiographic assessment also allows for evaluation of component positioning, with hip CT scan preferred. Infectious etiology must also be ruled out with appropriate lab work.

WORK UP

Physical examination should include both the lower extremities.

- Inspect for gross shortening or lengthening and lower extremity malrotation comparing to the contralateral limb.
- Palpate for step-off. Often, the femoral head can be palpated. A large palpable hematoma may indicates vascular injury.
- A neurovascular assessment of the full lower extremities is important to rule out important associated injuries. Pre-reduction neurovascular status must be carefully documented.
- Radiographic evaluation is important in determining direction of dislocation and component position (Figs 6.1A and B). Fluoroscopy can be used to examine for component loosening. A CT scan of the hip is preferable to determine component malposition.
- A lab workup to rule out infection should also be completed. This typically includes a CBC with differential, a C-reactive protein (CRP) level and erythrocyte sedimentation rate (ESR).

TREATMENT

Prompt closed reduction should be attempted regardless of the direction of dislocation if components are positioned well and there is no evidence for component failure. Successful reduction relies on adequate muscle relaxation achieved through the use of

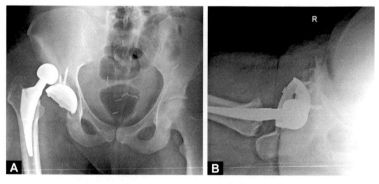

Figs 6.1A and B Showing evidence of a dislocated total hip arthroplasty of the right hip. (A) Anteroposterior view of the pelvis; (B) Cross table lateral view

sedation and analgesia and/or anesthesia. Care must be taken not to use excessive force or multiple attempts to reduce the dislocation as this can lead to prosthetic joint surface damage. Retrieval studies of implants that underwent open reductions after failure of repeated attempts at closed reduction showed significant macroscopic as well as microscopic damage to both metal and ceramic components.

Multiple techniques have been described to achieve reduction of the dislocated total hip replacement. With well-positioned components, the success rate for reduction subsequent to an early dislocation is high. Closed reduction may be attempted through the use of in-line traction while the patient is in a supine position on a locked stretcher. A first attempt should be made with conscious sedation; however, general anesthesia may be necessary to gain the appropriate level of relaxation.

■ The Allis Method

- Position the patient supine on a locked stretcher or table.
- The clinician stands above the patient on the stretcher.
- The clinician applies traction inline with the deformity while an assistant provides countertraction by stabilizing the patient's pelvis with both hands (Fig. 6.2A).

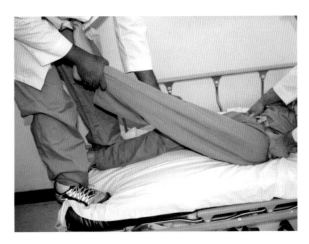

Fig. 6.2A Application of in-line traction while an assistant stabilizes the patient's pelvis with both hands

- As the clinician slowly increases force of traction, hip flexion is gently increased to 70 to 90° (Fig. 6.2B).
- Slight adduction and gentle rotational motions may help in achieving reduction, heralded by an audible "clunk" (Figs 6.2C and D).

The Bigelow Maneuver

- As in the Allis method, the patient is positioned supine.
- Longitudinal traction is applied by the clinician with an assistant stabilizing the pelvis for countertraction (Fig. 6.3A).
- The adducted and internally rotated thigh is flexed to 90° (Fig. 6.3B).
- Abduction results in reduction of the femoral head into the acetabulum (Fig. 6.3C).

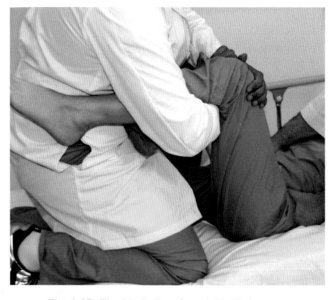

Fig. 6.2B The hip is then flexed 70-90 degrees

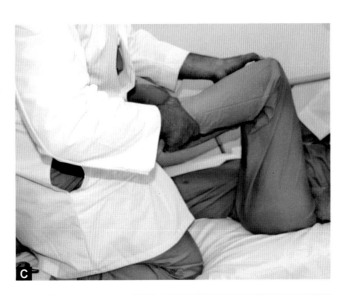

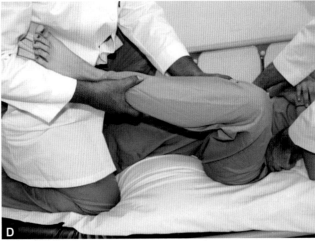

Figs 6.2C and D The addition of slight adduction and rotation facilitates reduction of the femoral head into the acetabulum

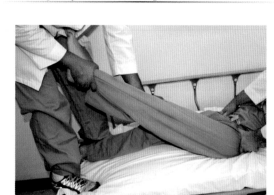

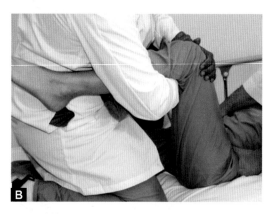

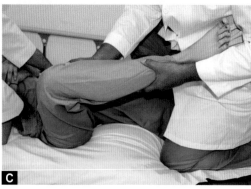

Figs 6.3A-C 90-90 traction can disengage the dislocated femoral head allowing slight abduction and rotation to reduce the femoral head

■ The Reverse Bigelow Maneuver

The reverse Bigelow maneuver method is used for anterior dislocations and comprises of following steps:

- The hip is adducted and internally rotated.
- The hip is slowly extended.

■ Stimson Technique (Gravity Method)

- Place the patient in a prone position with the affected leg hanging off the stretcher (Fig. 6.4).
- The hip and knee should both be flexed to 90°.
- An assistant should stabilize the pelvis while the surgeon applies anterior force to the proximal calf (Fig. 6.5).
- Reduction is often aided by gentle rotational movements of the hip.

POST-REDUCTION CARE

- Post-reduction films are important to confirm the success of the maneuver (Figs 6.6A-C). Fluoroscopy can be used, if available, to gauge stability of the joint. It is important to evaluate for laxity that could result in re-dislocation.

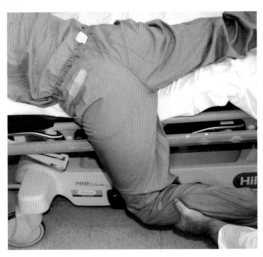

Fig. 6.4 Patient in a prone position with the affected leg hanging off the stretcher

Emergency Room Orthopaedic Procedures

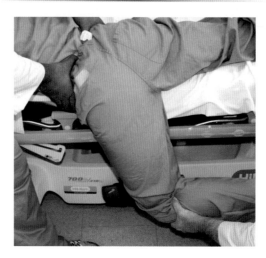

Fig. 6.5 The treating practitioner applies an anterior force to the proximal calf as an assistant stabilizes the pelvis with both hands

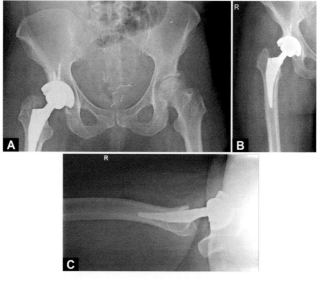

Figs 6.6A-C Post-reduction anteroposterior view of the pelvis, anteroposterior view of the right hip and cross table lateral view demonstrating successful reduction of the femoral head component into the acetabulum

- A careful neurovascular assessment is also necessary, as damage to the sciatic nerve is possible during hip reduction.
- There is disagreement over restrictions to weightbearing and range of motion. Typically, the patient is restricted from full weight bearing until free from pain.
- Immobilization also remains controversial. Abduction bracing, while common, has been shown recently to have limited impact on outcomes following closed treatment of THA dislocations[1]. Knee immobilization is another option which prevents patients from flexing the hip beyond a safe range.
- In some patients with cognitive impairment that would make adherence to ROM restriction difficult, a full length SPICA cast or hip immobilizer may be used, but this is often poorly tolerated in this patient population.

REFERENCE

1. Hargovind DeWal, Stephen L Maurer, Peter Tsai, et al. Efficacy of abduction bracing in the management of total hip arthroplasty dislocation. The Journal of Arthroplasty. 2004;19(6):733-8.

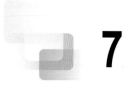

7

Insertion of Femoral and Tibial Traction Pins

Sonya Khurana, Eric J Strauss

INTRODUCTION

Skeletal traction is indicated for fractures and dislocations, mainly of the lower extremity. Skeletal traction using femoral or tibial traction pins provides reduction and temporary stabilization of pelvic, hip or femur injuries where splinting is not effective, acetabular fractures with or without concomitant hip dislocation, pelvic vertical shear injuries and shortened femoral shaft fractures.

Indications for insertion of distal femoral pins include some acetabular fractures most pelvic fractures with a displaced hemi-pelvis and most femoral shaft fractures.

Indications for insertion of proximal tibial traction pins include those for distal femur pins in cases where a soft tissue contra indication exists. Contraindications for placement of proximal tibial traction pins include ligamentous injury to the ipsilateral knee (check for swelling of knee after initial injury or when the patient is in traction), a patient who is skeletally immature (may cause recurvatum injury due to damage to the tibial physis), ipsilateral long stem TKA, and/or a tibial plateau fracture with metaphyseal comminution.

Risks of traction pin insertion include medullary canal contamination, neurovascular injury, potential intra-articular contamination, pin tract infection, fracture, generation of a stress-riser which can lead to subsequent fractures and heterotopic ossification within surrounding musculature.

It is important to insert the pin from the area of most risk to the area of least risk, as the direction of the pin can be controlled only during its insertion and the path cannot be altered once it exits bone. Distal femoral pins carry risk of injury to the superficial femoral artery in the adductor canal and thus should be inserted from the medial side toward the lateral side. Proximal tibial pins carry risk of injury to the peroneal nerve and anterior tibial artery and therefore should be inserted from the lateral side toward the medial side.

To place a traction pin, either a Kirschner wire or Steinmann pin is inserted bicortically through bone. Kirschner wires are smooth and cause less injury to soft tissues due to their smaller diameter. A tensioned traction bow must be used with the thin wire. Steinmann pins can be smooth, partially threaded, or fully threaded and are available in many sizes. The threaded pins are associated with a more traumatic insertion but are less likely to loosen or migrate over time compared with smooth pins. However, smooth pins are somewhat stronger than the threaded pins and are less likely to bend when traction is applied. Partially threaded pins are more difficult to insert than the threaded and smooth pins because the non-threaded portion is more difficult to advance through bone. In general, pin size is based on the diameter of the bone and the pin diameter should always be less than 30 percent of the diameter of the bone. Smaller smooth pins should be used in children with open physes.

In general, the pin should be placed parallel to the joint and in appropriate relation to the limb axis. Try to avoid placing the tibial pin into cortical bone more than 8 cm distal to the knee, as this is associated with an increased risk of tibia fractures. Avoid tension at the pin/skin interface. Avoid oblique pin placement in any plane.

MATERIALS REQUIRED

Materials required are Steinmann pin or Kirschner wire, hand drill power drill or wire driver, Jacob's chuck, soft tissue protection sleeve, bolt cutter, Steinmann pin or Kirschner wire holder, Xeroform and Webril.

STEPS

■ Distal Femoral Pins

- Ensure that the patient is adequately sedated.
- Position the patient supine on the ER table or operating table.

- Prepare and drape the thigh in a sterile manner.
- Locate the appropriate starting point two fingerbreadths proximal to the superior pole of the patella, a point just proximal to the adductor tubercle (Fig. 7.1).
- Inject a local anesthetic agent into the subcutaneous and subperiosteal tissue on the medial and lateral sides (Fig. 7.2).
- Using a 15 blade, make a short longitudinal incision just proximal to the adductor tubercle, medial epicondyle and/or growth

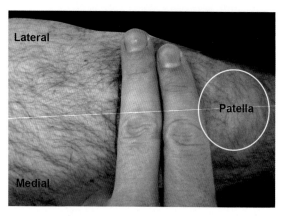

Fig. 7.1 The appropriate starting point for a distal femoral traction pin is identified, two fingerbreadths proximal to the superior pole of the patella

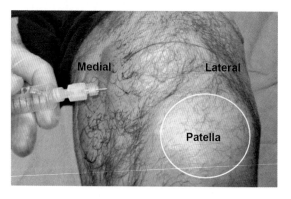

Fig. 7.2 After prepping the medial aspect of the distal femur with povidone-iodine, the site of the traction pin starting point is injected with local anesthetic

plate. After the knife is buried, underneath the skin, turn it to 90°
to make a small nick in the iliotibial band (Fig. 7.3).

- Insert a 3/16 inch Steinmann pin or 1.6 mm or 2.0 mm Kirschner
  wire using a hand drill of power drill (Fig 7.4). The pin or K-wire
  should be inserted parallel to the joint line.

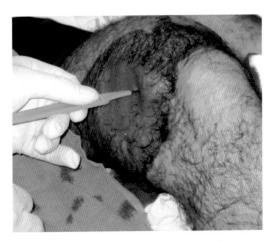

Fig. 7.3 Making a short longitudinal incision just proximal to
the adductor tubercle, medial epicondyle and/or growth plate

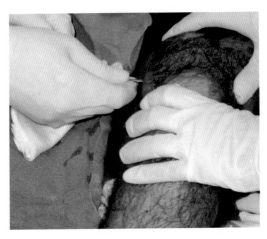

Fig. 7.4 Insertion of 3/16 inch Steinmann pin from medial to lateral,
parallel to the knee joint line

- Palpate the pin as it exits the far lateral cortex and make a skin incision over this area to permit passage of the pin (Figs 7.5A and B).
- Apply xeroform/Vaseline dressing followed by a gauze wrap.
- Cut the ends of the inserted traction pin with a bolt cutter and apply the appropriate traction bow. When Steinmann pins or thick K-wires are used a standard traction bow is utilized. For smaller diameter K-wires, a tension bow is used (Figs 7.6 and 7.7)

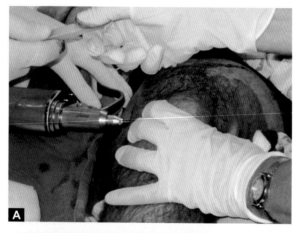

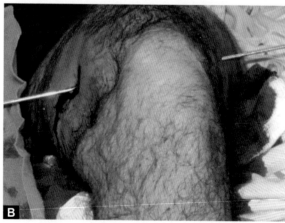

Figs 7.5A and B (A) The tip of the pin or K-wire is felt on the lateral aspect of the thigh. After injecting this site with local anesthetic a small incision is made in the skin; (B) to permit passage

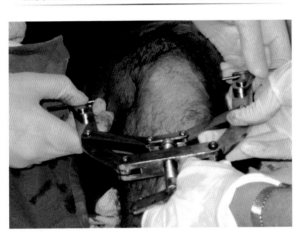

Fig. 7.6 Application of the traction bow to the inserted traction pin

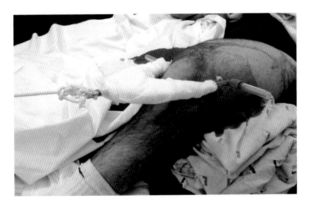

Fig. 7.7 Application of traction to the traction pin-traction bow set up. Test tubes may be placed over the sharp pin ends to prevent injury to the patient or the healthcare provider

- Place the patient into the appropriate traction (approximately 15% of his or her body weight). Flex the affected knee to 20 to 30° for balanced skeletal traction or to 90° for 90-90 traction (Fig. 7.8). A bump should be placed underneath the knee to facilitate this.
- Take X-rays to ensure proper pin placement if unsure of placement and limb alignment No weight should be applied until one is certain of the pins position within the bone.

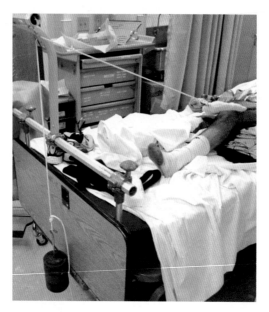

Fig. 7.8 Proper set up of balanced distal femoral traction with the knee in 20-30° of flexion and 1/10 of the patient's body weight applied using a pulley system attached to the end of the bed

■ Proximal Tibial Pins

- Ensure that the patient is adequately sedated.
- Position the patient supine on the ER table or operating table.
- Flex the knee to 20 to 30° (or the degree needed for flexion) using a bump.
- Prep and drape the leg in a sterile manner.
- Inject a local anesthetic agent into the subcutaneous and subperiosteal tissue on the medial and lateral sides.
- A vertical incision at the level of the tibial tubercle should be made approximately 1 to 2 cm anterior to the anterior border of the fibular head and just below the tibial tuberosity on the lateral side of the tibia.
- Using a hemostat, bluntly dissect to the lateral tibial cortex.
- Insert a 3/16 inch Steinmann pin or thick Kirschner wire using a hand drill of power drill (Fig. 7.4). The pin or K-wire should be inserted parallel to the joint line.
- Palpate the pin as it exits the far medial cortex and make a skin incision over this area to allow for passage of the pin.

- Apply xeroform/Vaseline dressing followed by a gauze wrap.
- Trim the ends of the pin with a bolt cutter and attach a Steinmann pin holder or Kirschner wire holder to the traction pin.
- Place the patient into the appropriate traction (approximately 15% of his or her body weight).
- Take X-rays to ensure proper pin placement and limb alignment as previously described.

SUGGESTED READINGS

1. Althausen PL, Hak DK. Lower extremity traction pins: indications, technique and complications. Am J Orthop (Belle Mead NJ). 2002; 3. 31(1):43-7.
2. Kwon, et al. Lateral femoral traction pin entry: risk to the femoral artery and other medial neurovascular structures. J Orthop Surg Res. 2010;5:4.
3. Merk Bradley R. Femoral and tibial traction pin placement. In: Stern, Steven H (Eds). Key Techniques in Orthopaedic Surgery. NewYork: Thieme; 2001. pp. 321-5.
4. Wheeless III, Clifford R. Femoral and tibial traction pins. Wheeless' Textbook of Orthopaedics; 2010.
5. World Health Organization Traction. Essential Surgical Care Manual [online]. Available from <http://www.steinergraphics.com/surgical/006_17.1.html>. Accessed March 2011.

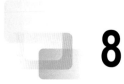

8

The Evaluation and Management of Nursemaid's Elbow

Robert C Rothberg

INTRODUCTION

Nursemaid's elbow, or "pulled elbow" of childhood occurs when an axial traction (distracting) force is applied to an abducted arm with the elbow in extension and pronation, resulting in a tear of the incompletely developed annular ligament in children.

Traditionally, a subluxation of the radial head[18] (the entity's other name) was thought to result directly but cadaver studies performed by Hutchinson and Salter describe a more complex process. As the radius subluxes inferiorly and anteriorly due to the applied traction, a tear of the most distal insertion of the annular ligament on the radial neck occurs. This results in a subluxation of the partially torn annular ligament superiorly, exposing the anterior portion of the radial head. The torn segment of the annular ligament becomes interposed in the joint space between the radial head and capitellum.[4,12] Pronation is a prerequisite along with elbow extension for this injury to be produced; it will not occur in supination.[5,14] The classic situations in which this mechanism results in the nursemaid injury occur when a child is being pulled by the wrist by a caregiver and the child either resists or falls, or by picking up or swinging a child by the arms.

Nursemaid's elbow typically occurs in children less than 5 years old, with a range from as young as 3 months[8] to 73 months.[15] The peak age for occurrence is approximately 26 months.[8,12,15] However, this injury has also been described in adolescence[9] and in at least one instance as an isolated injury (not as part of a Monteggia injury pattern) in an adult patient.[11]

Nursemaid's elbow is a common pediatric injury, representing approximately 20 percent of upper extremity injuries.[12] On presentation, the classic mechanism of a pulling injury has been reported to be present in 51 to 93 percent of cases.[12,15] More typically, a non-classic mechanism is elicited in one-third of cases.[13] Other reported mechanisms offered by parents have included falls (22% reported by Schunk;[15] 7% reported by Quan[12]) or unknown mechanism (20% reported by Schunk[15]). In children less than six months old, a common alternative mechanism is rolling over or being assisted in rolling over.[8] A possible contributing factor involved in some of the non-classic mechanisms reported may be due to reluctance on the part of caregivers to accurately describe what occurred due to issues of responsibility for contributing to the injury.

Caregivers usually report that at the time of the injury, the child suddenly started crying for a variable period of time followed by a refusal to move the injured extremity. However, caregivers are frequently unable to localize the level of the injury on the affected arm. In the study by Quan[12] that looked at presenting chief complaints of patients ultimately found to have a nursemaid's elbow injury, elbow injury was only recorded 10 percent of the time. Other chief complaints included: arm injury (61%), shoulder injury (10%), sprain (11%), and wrist injury (4%).

There is a slight predilection for involvement of the left arm (61% reported by Schunk,[15] 58% by McDonald[8] and 57% by Teach[19]) which is postulated to result from the fact that most caregivers are right handed and would therefore be expected to favor grasping the patient's left hand with their right hand.[12]

PHYSICAL EXAMINATION

At the time of examination, the pediatric patient is usually not experiencing active pain but is observed not to move the affected arm and cannot be coaxed to use it with offers of a toy or food (Fig. 8.1). The elbow should look uninjured (no gross deformities) but still (no spontaneous movements). The classic attitude of the injured extremity (referred to as the nursemaid's position), is one of adduction, with flexion at the elbow and partial pronation.

What will be absent on inspection is any degree of supination which is a clue to the diagnosis. There should also be no observed swelling and no ecchymosis.

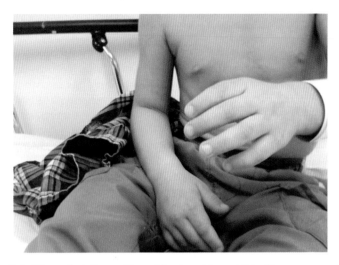

Fig. 8.1 Characteristic position of the hand in a child with a nursemaid's elbow. The patient is hesitant to move the injured upper extremity

On palpation, tenderness may be elicited over the radial head but none should be found over the distal humerus, olecranon or proximal ulna. Limited passive range of motion for flexion and extension may be tolerated by the patient but typically supination will be resisted and will frequently elicit crying.

Assessment of the neurovascular status should be performed including documentation of normal motor function for the anterior interosseus nerve ("OK" sign with thumb and index finger), posterior interosseus nerve ("Hitchhikers" sign with thumb extension) and ulnar nerve ("Crossed finger" sign, ability of middle finger to cross dorsally over index finger) and sensory function of the radial nerve (first dorsal webspace), median nerve (volar pad of index finger), and ulnar nerve (volar pad of small finger). Documentation of the presence of radial and ulnar pulses and adequacy of capillary refill should be recorded.

Standard radiographs of the elbow (AP, lateral and oblique) are typically negative for abnormal findings.[16] Classically, this has been explained by the fact that although the radial head subluxes inferiorly and anteriorly due to the distracting force that occurs during the injury, the radial head then spontaneously reduces and therefore, no radiographic abnormality should be expected. It is for these reasons that radiographic imaging is felt not to be indicated when the suspicion is high for a nursemaid's elbow injury. However, two reports describe abnormalities involving the radiocapitellar line (normally a line drawn through the center of the proximal humerus should always bisect the middle-third of the humeral capitellum on any view) on X-rays obtained in patients ultimately determined to have nursemaid's elbow injuries.[2,17] Both the studies described displacement of the radiocapitellar line off the capitellum.

Approach to the Child with a Suspected Nursemaid's Elbow

Scenario 1

- The history is consistent with a nursemaid's elbow mechanism of injury.
- The arm is in the nursemaid's position.
- At most, only mild tenderness is localized over the radial head without elbow swelling or ecchymosis.
- Recommendation: Elbow radiographs are not indicated and it is acceptable to proceed directly to reduction.[12] The hyperpronation technique is the recommended first technique to employ.

Scenario 2

- History is unclear (either not witnessed by caregiver or non-standard mechanism).
- The arm is in the nursemaid's position.
- Tenderness is limited to the radial head (no distal humeral, olecranon, proximal ulna tenderness), no elbow swelling or ecchymosis.
- Controversial: Some authors recommend radiographs first, to rule out possibility of supracondylar fracture with the attendant risk of fracture displacement resulting from attempted nursemaid reduction maneuver.[7] Other authors noting the high incidence of atypical histories state, it is acceptable to proceed without X-rays first as long as no "atypical" physical findings are present (point tenderness was included as an atypical feature).[17]
- Recommendation: In the setting of witnessed or suspected fall onto the elbow or outstretched hand, it is prudent to obtain

radiographs first to rule out fracture. Otherwise, it is acceptable to proceed directly with a reduction attempt without first obtaining elbow radiographs, adhering to the caveat that at most minimal tenderness limited to the radial head may be present, but the presence of tenderness at other locations, elbow swelling, or ecchymosis should prompt radiographic evaluation before attempted reduction.

Scenario 3

- History is unclear or non-standard mechanism.
- Any of the following findings are present: swelling, ecchymosis, or tenderness over distal humerus, humeral condyles, olecranon, proximal ulna.
- Recommendation requires radiographic imaging first to rule out an osseous injury, in particular a supracondylar fracture.

■ Reduction Maneuvers for Nursemaid's Elbow

Supination-flexion involves supination at the wrist followed by flexion at the elbow.[1,3,8,10,12,15] This has been the standard reduction technique with which most physicians are familiar.

The technique is as follows:

- The thumb of the examiner is placed over the radial head of the patient's affected arm. The examiner then grasps the patient's wrist with the other hand (Fig. 8.2).
- The patient's elbow is passively positioned at 90° of flexion.
- The examiner then actively supinates the patient's wrist to 90° in one steady movement, followed by actively flexing the patient's elbow to maximal flexion (Figs 8.3 and 8.4). During this two-step maneuver, a palpable (or possibly audible) click should be elicited.

An alternative technique is the pronation or hyperpronation technique (with or without flexion).[1,3,8] This technique was originally described as the preferred method of reduction by Hutchinson.[4,5] The version of this technique, that is recommended is a variation on the "handshake" described by Lyver.[6]

The technique is as follows:

- The thumb of the examiner is again placed over the radial head of the patient's affected arm.

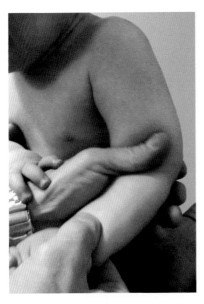

Fig. 8.2 Placing the thumb of the examiner over the radial head of the patient's affected arm while performing reduction technique

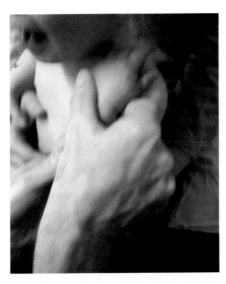

Fig. 8.3 Supination of the patient's wrist to 90° in one steady movement, followed by actively flexing the patient's elbow to maximal flexion

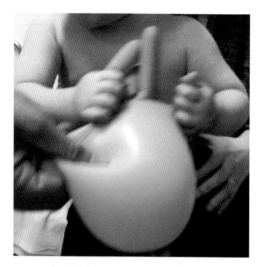

Fig. 8.4 Following successful reduction the patient now actively uses the upper extremity indicating resolution of symptoms

- The examiner then grasps the patients hand in a handshake with the examiner's other hand (Fig. 8.5).
- The examiner then actively pronates the patients hand until a palpable or audible click is elicited (Fig. 8.6).

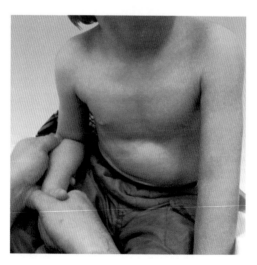

Fig. 8.5 Examiner grasping the patient's hand in a handshake

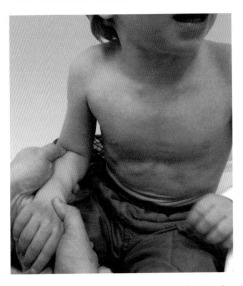

Fig. 8.6 Examiner pronating the patient's hand until a
palpable or audible click is elicited

- If no click is appreciated by 90° of pronation, the patient's hand
  is maximally hyperpronated (Fig. 8.7). Mild flexion can be added
  to hyperpronation, although this is usually not necessary.

Several prospective studies have compared the two techniques.
McDonald[8] found equal success rates between the two maneuvers but found hyperpronation more successful when the left arm

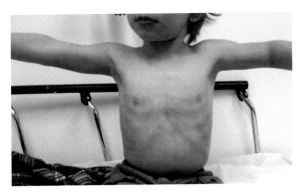

Fig. 8.7 Actively uses the upper extremity indicating
resolution of symptoms

was involved and was judged to be less painful by the clinicians performing the procedure. The author concluded by recommending the pronation technique as the favored maneuver. Bek[1] more recently found equal final reduction rates but that hyperpronation was more likely to result in reduction on the first attempt, associated with less pain for the patient and easier to perform by the clinician. He similarly recommended hyperpronation as the "first choice" for reducing nursemaid elbow injuries.

The occurrence of a palpable or audible click indicates that the annular ligament has been reduced with either technique.[4,14] The child will usually cry briefly at the time of reduction, followed by full use of the affected arm within 30 minutes. A second attempt should be made with the same technique if reduction is not achieved on the first attempt. If the second attempt is unsuccessful, then the alternate technique should be attempted, and if not successful on the first attempt, a second attempt may be performed. If reduction is not then achieved, a plaster posterior splint should be applied with referral in several days to a pediatric orthopedist for follow-up.

DISCHARGE PLANS FOLLOWING SUCCESSFUL REDUCTION

The caregivers should be informed that a recurrent nursemaid's elbow is a possibility until complete development of the distal attachment of the annual ligament to the radial neck occurs usually by age 5.[14] It is acceptable to instruct the caregivers in the reduction technique that led to successful reduction so that they may attempt it prior to seeking medical care. In addition, it is reasonable to review the mechanism producing the injury with the caregivers and recommend avoiding the activity that resulted in the injury if at all possible. Applying a splint or sling for a patient fully using the affected arm after reduction is unnecessary and not recommended even in the setting of a recurrent nursemaid's dislocation, which has a reported frequency as high as 25 percent.[15,19]

REFERENCES

1. Bek D. Pronation versus supination maneuvers for the reduction of 'pulled elbow': a randomized clinical trial. 2009;16(3):135-8.
2. Frumkin K. Nursemaid's elbow: a radiographic demonstration. Annals of Emergency Medicine. 1985;14(7):690-3.

3. Green DA. Randomized comparison of pain perception during radial head subluxation reduction using supination-flexion or forced pronation. Pediatric Emergency Care. 2006;22(4):235-8.

4. Hutchinson J. On certain obscure sprains of the elbow occurring in young children. Annals of Surgery.1885;2:91-8.

5. Hutchinson J. Partial dislocation of the head of the radius peculiar to children. British Medical Journal. 1886;1:9-10.

6. Lyver M. Radial head subluxation [letter]. Journal of Emergency Medicine. 1990;8:154-5.

7. Mayeda D. A little smile [editorial]. Journal of Emergency Medicine.1990;8:203.

8. McDonald J. Radial head subluxation: comparing two methods of reduction. Academic Emergency Medicine. 1999;6(7):715-8.

9. Miller T. Radial head subluxation in adolescence. NY State Journal of Medicine. 1975;75:80-2.

10. Newman J. "Nursemaid's elbow" in infants six months and under. Journal of Emergency Medicine. 1985;2:403-4.

11. Pearson B. Nursemaid's elbow in a 31 year old female. American Journal of Emergency Medicine. 2006;6:222-3.

12. Quan L. The epidemiology and treatment of radial head subluxation. American Journal of Diseases of Children. 1985;139:1194-7.

13. Sacchetti A. Nonclassic history in children with radial head subluxation. 1990;8:151-3.

14. Salter R. Anatomic investigations of the mechanism of injury and pathologic anatomy of "pulled elbow" in young children. Clinical Orthopedics and Related Research. 1971;77:134-43.

15. Schunk J. Radial head subluxation: epidemiology and treatment of 87 episodes. 1990;19(9):1019-23.

16. Snyder H. Radiographic changes with radial head subluxation in children. Journal of Emergency Medicine. 1990;8:265-9.

17. Snyder H. Response from Dr Synder [letter]. Journal of Emergency Medicine. 1990;8:155-6.

18. Stone C. Subluxation of the head of the radius. JAMA. 1916;67(1):28-9.

19. Teach S. Prospective study of recurrent radial head subluxation. Arch Pediatr Adolescent Medicine. 1996;150:164-6.

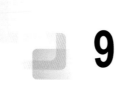

9

Closed Reduction of Distal Radius Fractures

Colin Prensky, Kenneth A Egol

INTRODUCTION

The distal radius accounts for approximately 15 to 20 percent of all fractures. About half of these are intra-articular injuries. Typically, distal radius fractures have a bimodal distribution, affecting children and the elderly. Distal radius fracture usually results from a fall on an outstretched arm. High energy injuries such as motor vehicle accidents or high-speed recreational activities like snowboarding are more likely to lead to open fractures.

The majority of distal radius fractures can be successfully treated with nonsurgical management. Fractures with stable metaphyseal support and minimal displacement can be treated with immobilization of the wrist with a cast or splint. Unstable fractures will often slip to their pre-reduction position and are poor candidates for closed management. Regular follow-up to monitor for proper radiographic alignment is recommended.

Good functional outcomes rely heavily on good anatomic reduction of the fracture, especially when the injury has an intra-articular component. Recent clinical studies have demonstrated that articular surface incongruities are the most important predictors of functional outcome, with restoration of radial length and volar tilt also influencing results.

HISTORY AND PHYSICAL EXAMINATION

The patient usually describes a fall or direct trauma to the wrist, with associated pain and/or gross deformity. While asking questions related to the patient's mechanism of injury, the physician should also be sure to inquire about any history of previous injuries or surgery to the forearm that may lead to anatomical variation. Carpal tunnel syndrome, peripheral vascular disease and rheumatoid arthritis are important relevant medical conditions.

The clinician must first determine whether the fracture is open or closed. In the case of an open fracture, treatment must be made on an emergent basis. The physician should examine the area for evidence of gross deformity, swelling, ecchymosis or open fracture. It is possible for the extremity to appear grossly normal if swelling has not had time to occur. The classic "dinner-fork" deformity commonly associated with Colles' fracture may also be present. The physician should carefully palpate for the area of maximal tenderness, examining for cortical step-off that demonstrates appreciable displacement. Scaphoid fracture may be ruled out with ulnar deviation and palpation of the anatomic snuffbox. The ipsilateral elbow should also be examined, with careful attention paid to potential associated injuries.

Careful assessment and documentation of neurovascular status before attempting any intervention is extremely important. As the median nerve is often compressed with displacement of the fracture, attention should be paid to sensation of the palmar aspect of the thumb and index finger. Compromise to neurovascular status is an indication for the attempt of immediate closed reduction. If possible, range of motion should also be evaluated.

■ Evaluation of Open Distal Radius Fractures

If the patient is medically stable, suspected open fractures must be carefully evaluated and treated emergently in the operating room.

- Examine the wound for signs of gross contamination. Studies have shown that the degree of wound contamination has the greatest effect on infection risk, while time to debridement does not.
- Debride the wound of any devitalized tissue and copiously irrigate the wound.

- It is recommended that the fracture be reduced and/or stabilized early in the emergency room, with definitive surgical treatment to be done when any life-threatening conditions that may have resulted from the original trauma have been addressed.

Radiographic Evaluation

High-quality radiographs are extremely important in order to properly evaluate the fracture and establish a treatment plan. True postero-anterior and lateral views are always obtained (Figs 9.1A-C). Often oblique view films are used to supplement the first two.

A radiographic evaluation is complete when it can address several key concerns.

- The clinician should assess for a loss of normal anatomy through angulation, displacement, impaction, etc.
- The next concern is whether the fracture involves the radiocarpal or distal radioulnar joint. If a joint is involved, the physician must note whether there exists discontinuity or separation of the artic-ular surface.
- Finally, high-risk features such as severe comminution, articular step-off greater than 2 mm or fracture-dislocation are good indications for considering surgical intervention.
- The contralateral wrist views may be useful in determining the patient's normal ulnar variance and scapholunate angle. Figures 9.2A-C for normal values.

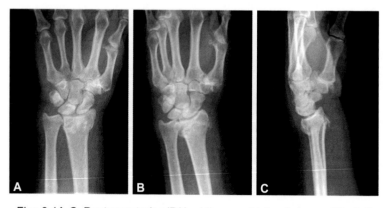

Figs 9.1A-C Posteroanterior (PA), oblique and lateral views of the left wrist showing evidence of a displaced distal radius fracture

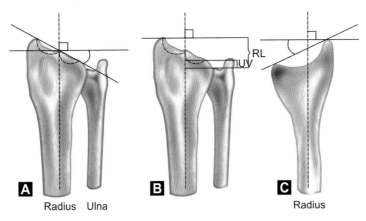

Figs 9.2A-C (A) Radial inclination; (B) Radial shortening; and (C) Volar tilt

Radial inclination: 13–30°
Radial length: 8–18 mm
Volar tilt: 0–28°

Significant displacement of the articular surface greater than 1–2 mm, angulation of more than 20°, shortening by more than 3 mm and acute median nerve compression, all are indications for reduction.

Technique of Closed Reduction and Splint Immobilization

Materials

A 3- or 4-inch plaster, 4- or 4-inch webril, basin with lukewarm water, 10 cc syringe, 1% lidocaine, skin prep, fingertraps and traction weights are required (Fig. 9.3).

- Prepare a syringe with 10 ml of 0.5% lidocaine for hematoma block (Fig. 9.4).
- Prepare the overlying skin with povidone-iodine or chlorhexidine and inject anesthetic directly into fracture site (Figs 9.5 and 9.6). Confirm location by looking for blood flashback from the hematoma.

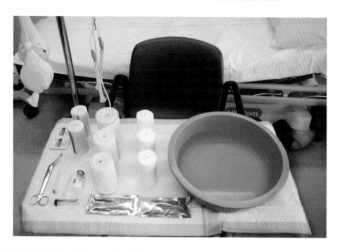

Fig. 9.3 Materials needed for reduction and splint immobilization of distal radius fractures

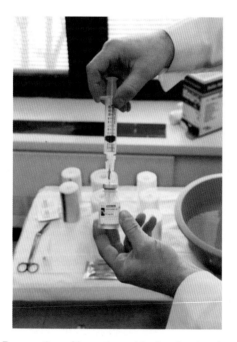

Fig. 9.4 Preparation of hematoma block using local anesthetic (1% lidocaine without epinephrine)

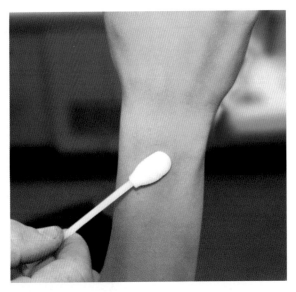

Fig. 9.5 Application of povidone-iodine or chlorhexidine over the dorsal aspect of the wrist for the hematoma block

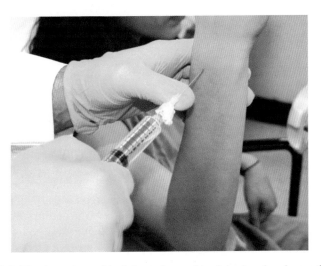

Fig. 9.6 The hematoma block is performed by injecting local anesthetic directly into the fracture site. A flashback of blood confirms appropriate localization of the hematoma block

- Apply traction to the injured wrist using finger traps and 5–10 lbs of weight from the patient's arm proximal to the elbow as shown in Figure 9.7.
- Allow at least 5 to 10 minutes of traction for adequate muscle relaxation and bony fragment disengagement.
- While traction is being applied, prepare casting materials (Fig. 9.8).
- With finger traps still in place, the physician positions his or her thumbs on the distal fragment (Fig. 9.9). The physician's fingers are positioned on the radius, directly distal to the fracture line (Fig 9.10).
- While longitudinal traction distracts the bone fragments, the physician's thumbs manipulate the distal fragment into anatomic position, assuring proper alignment and length. Avoid positions of extreme wrist flexion due to the complication of median nerve compression. If such positions are necessary to maintain reduction, surgical fixation may be necessary.

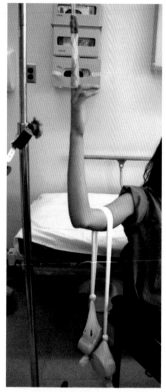

Fig. 9.7 Reduction is assisted by using traction with finger traps and weights hung on the patient's suspended upper arm

- Wrap the hand and wrist with one layer of cotton webril, maintaining proper positioning of the wrist to prevent re-displacement (Figs 9.11A and B).
- After placing the cotton webril, repeat steps 6 and 7 to ensure that the fracture fragment has not slipped. The cotton webril has some "memory" and will provide some degree of support for the wrist positioning.
- Wrap a second layer of cotton web roll (Fig. 9.12).
- Measure out the plaster extending from the level of the metacarpophalangeal joints dorsally to the palmar flexion crease (Fig. 9.13).

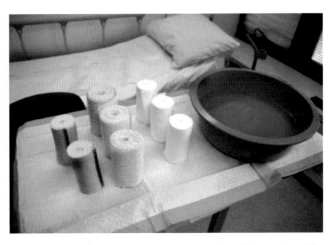

Fig. 9.8 Materials needed for splint immobilization of the reduced fracture

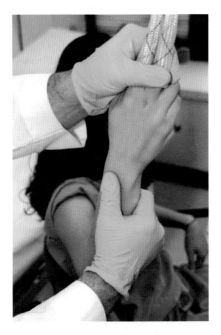

Fig. 9.9 Reduction maneuver with the physician's thumb placed on the distal fracture fragment and the other hand restoring radial height and inclination

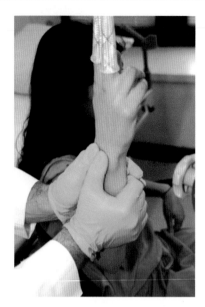

Fig. 9.10 The distal fracture fragment is reduced with the physician's
thumbs pressing from a dorsal to volar direction

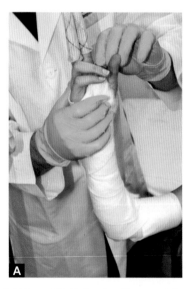 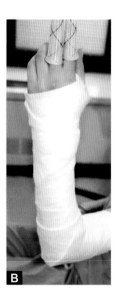

Figs 9.11A and B Following the provisional reduction the patient's hand
an wrist are wrapped with 2-3 layers of webril cotton undercast padding.
Care is taken to pad the bony olecranon process

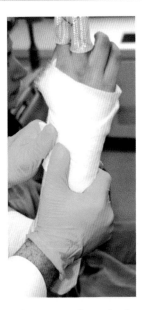

Fig. 9.12 The physician's repeats the reduction maneuver once the webril layers are applied

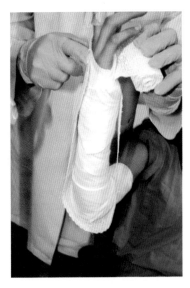

Fig. 9.13 Measuring out the plaster for the splint extending from the level of the metacarpophalangeal (MCP) joints dorsally to the palmar flexion crease volarly

- Apply a well-molded sugar-tong splint to the patient's wrist and hand, ensuring freedom of movement of the metacarpophalangeal joints (Figs 9.14A and B, and 9.15A to D). A neutral or slightly palmar-flexed wrist position is preferred.
- After swelling has subsided, a well molded cast may be used in place of the sugar-tong splint.

POST REDUCTION CARE

- Radiographic evaluation immediately following splinting is necessary to ensure adequate reduction.
- Follow-up with repeat X-rays in 7 to 10 days is recommended to confirm no change in fracture fragment position.
- If the fracture shows re-displacement, it should be considered unstable and operative management is typically recommended with fixation by open reduction and internal fixation, percutaneous pins or ex fix (Figs 9.16 A and B).
- Immobilization in a cast or wrist splint is maintained for six weeks or until radiographs demonstrate evidence of bony union.

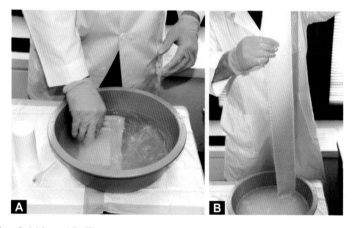

Figs 9.14A and B The plaster is dipped into lukewarm water and excess water is wrung out of the splint material

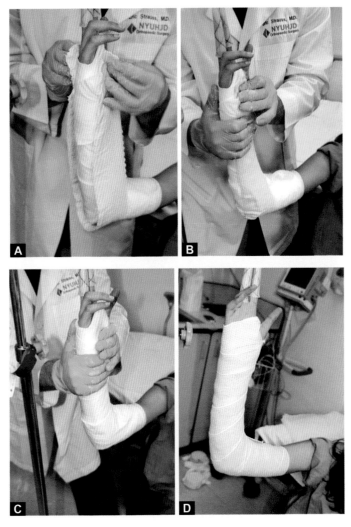

Figs 9.15A-D Application of a well-molded sugar-tong splint to the patient's wrist and hand

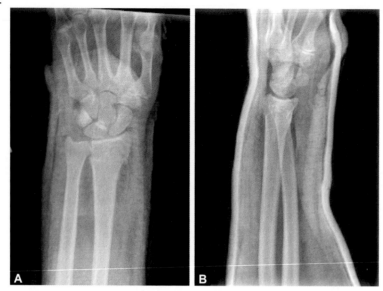

Figs 9.16A and B Post-reduction anteroposterior (AP) and lateral X-rays are taken to confirm adequate fracture fragment position

SUGGESTED READINGS

■ Textbook Chapters

1. Putnam M, Steitz W. "Fractures of the distal radius". Rockwood and Green's Fractures in Adults. Chapter 20:815-69.

■ Review Articles

1. Lichtman DM, Bindra RR, Boyer MI, et al. Treatment of distal radius fractures. J Am Acad Ortho Surg. 2010;18:180-9.
2. Liporace FA, Adams MR, Capo JT, et al. Distal radius fractures. J Orthop Trauma. 2009;23(10):739-48. Review.
3. Chen NC, Jupiter JB. Management of distal radial fractures. J Bone Joint Surg Am. 2007;89(9):2051-62. Review.

■ Relevant Studies

1. Egol KA, Walsh M, Romo-Cardoso S, et al. Distal radial fractures in the elderly: operative compared with nonoperative treatment. J Bone Joint Surg Am. 2010;92(9):1851-7.

2. Mackenney PJ, McQueen MM. Prediction of instability in distal radial fractures. J Bone Joint Surg Am. 2006;88(9):1944-51.

3. Rozental TD, Blazar PE. Functional outcome and complications after volar plating for dorsally displaced, unstable fractures of the distal radius. J Hand Surg Am. 2006;31(3):359-65.

4. Trumble TE, Schmitt SR. Factors affecting functional outcome of displaced intra-articular distal radius fractures. J Hand Surg Am. 1994;19(2):325-40.

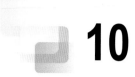

10

Nail Bed Repair

Eric J Strauss

INTRODUCTION

Fingertip injuries, especially those affecting the nail bed, are among the most common traumatic conditions presenting to emergency departments. Proper evaluation and management of these injuries is important in an effort to prevent long-term cosmetic and functional disability. Removal of the nail plate and inspection of the injury coupled with careful nail bed repair has proven to be the treatment of choice, offering the affected patient the best opportunity for a good outcome. Historically, meticulous repair of nail bed lacerations using fine, absorbable suture was the gold standard for management. Recent data has supported the use of 2-octylcyanoacrylate (Dermabond) as an alternative treatment approach, leading to equivalent cosmetic and functional results.

EMERGENCY ROOM EVALUATION

Upon presentation, the evaluating healthcare practitioner should obtain a complete history including the patient's hand dominance, occupation, past medical history, medication allergies and tetanus status. Details of the injury should also be sought, including the time of the injury and its mechanism, as crush or avulsion injuries often portend a worse prognosis than isolated nail bed lacerations.

The physical examination should ideally be performed prior to performing a digital nerve block, allowing for a complete assessment of the digit's neurovascular status. For patients in severe pain or in pediatric patients with nail bed injuries, the digital block may become necessary to allow a proper examination to proceed. The normal anatomy of the distal fingertip is shown in Figure 10.1. The gross appearance of the distal finger tip should be noted and documented including the presence of a subungual hematoma, injury to the surrounding skin, whether or not the nail plate is injured or intact and the overall posture of the digit indicating the possibility of an underlying distal phalanx fracture (present in 50% of nail bed injuries). A thorough neurovascular examination should be performed, evaluating sensation on both the sides of the injured finger tip in addition to the status of each digital artery. Depending on patient's comfort level, active range of motion can be assessed to rule out an associated flexor or extensor tendon injury.

Radiographic evaluation of the injured finger includes anteroposterior (AP), lateral and oblique views to identify associated distal phalanx fractures, distal interphalangeal (DIP) joint dislocations and whether or not any foreign bodies are present associated with the injury.

Once the overall condition of the finger is evaluated and X-rays are obtained, a digital nerve block followed by nail plate removal will allow further examination of the injured nail bed, classification of the injury (simple versus stellate laceration) and appropriate treatment to be performed.

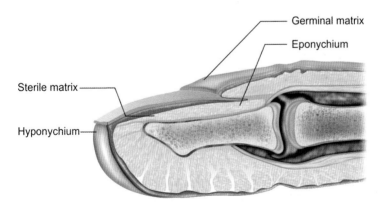

Fig. 10.1 Normal anatomy of the distal fingertip

TREATMENT OF NAIL BED INJURIES

Management of nail bed injuries will be dictated by the extent of the injury, the type of laceration present and the presence of associated pathology. Small subungual hematomas (those involving <25% of the nail bed) can be managed with observation or trephination, if the area is painful. For subungual hematomas involving more than 25% of the nail bed, nail plate removal is recommended for examination of the nail bed and repair of any laceration that may be present. Treatment options for both simple and stellate nail bed lacerations include suture repair or the use of 2-octylcyanoacrylate (Dermabond). Typically associated distal phalanx tuft fractures do not need specific management as nail bed repair will often reduce these injuries and allow them to heal.

■ Necessary Supplies for Nail Bed Repair

Materials required for nail bed repair are shown in Figure 10.2 and described as follows:

- 1% lidocaine without epinephrine for digital nerve block
- 10 cc syringe
- 25- or 27-gauge needle for the digital nerve block
- 0.5" or 1" penrose drain to act as a finger tourniquet
- Povidone-iodine solution
- Kidney basin

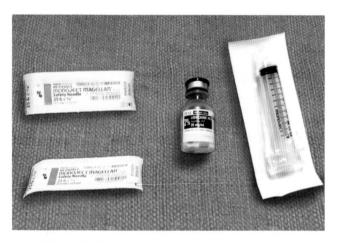

Fig. 10.2 Materials needed for digital nerve block

- Sterile drapes
- Laceration tray—necessary instruments include iris scissors, small needle driver, forceps and a small tissue elevator
- 6-0 absorbable monofilament suture
- 6-0 nylon suture (keep the foil package to use as an interposition underneath the eponychial fold if the patient's nail is unavailable or unusable)
- 2-octylcyanoacrylate (Dermabond, if this treatment approach is utilized)
- Xeroform non-adherent dressing
- Sterile dressings (gauze and kling wrap)
- Finger splint
- Loupe magnification (optional).

Technique: Suture Repair and 2-Octylcyanoacrylate Repair

With the patient in supine position, the affected hand is placed palm down onto an arm extension or small mayo stand type table. The injured finger is copiously irrigated with saline removing any debris or contamination from the region of the nail. The finger is then prepped using povidone-iodine solution and the area is draped using a sterile extremity drape. A digital nerve block is then provided making sure to cover all four digital nerves that supply the injured finger. The penrose drain is then applied as a finger tourniquet, wrapped from distal to proximal and anchored around the base of the finger. The nail plate is then removed and the nature of the nail bed laceration is assessed.

Digital Nerve Block

- Insert the needle perpendicular to the finger and into the subcutaneous tissue of the web space just distal to the metacarpophalangeal joint (Figs 10.3A and B).
- Slowly aspirate to ensure that the needle is not in a digital blood vessel.
- Inject 2 ml of anesthetic into the subcutaneous dorsal tissue, infiltrating the tissues around the dorsal nerve.
- Slowly advance the needle towards the palmar surface and inject an additional 2 ml of anesthetic as the needle goes along. This should infiltrate the tissues surrounding the palmar nerve do not push through the palmar skin surface.

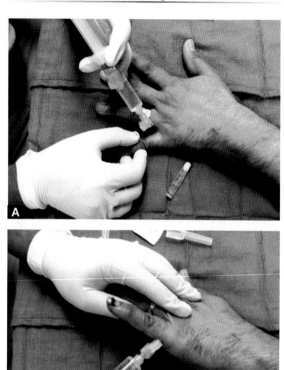

Figs 10.3A and B Digital nerve block is performed by injecting local anesthetic perpendicular to the finger both medially and laterally to anesthetize the radial and ulnar digital nerves

- Withdraw the needle and repeat these steps on the opposite side of the finger. Use 2 ml of anesthetic per nerve (for 8 ml total).

Nail Plate Removal

- Using the iris scissors placed between the nail bed and the nail plate (hyponchium), the nail plate is systematically released, opening and closing the tips of the scissors to provide tissue separation (Figs 10.4A and B).

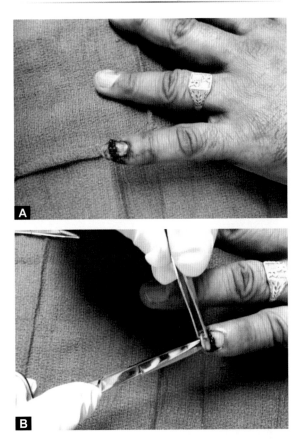

Figs 10.4A and B Nail plate removal using the iris scissors placed between the nail bed and the nail plate

- The iris scissors are advanced proximally until they reach the nail fold—making sure to free the nail plate proximally, radially and ulnarly.
- Once removed from the underlying nail bed, the nail plate should be saved for later interposition underneath the eponychial fold (place in kidney basin soaking in povidone-iodine).

Suture Repair

- Irrigate the nail bed removing any hematoma or debris (Fig. 10.5).
- Classify the laceration as either simple or stellate.

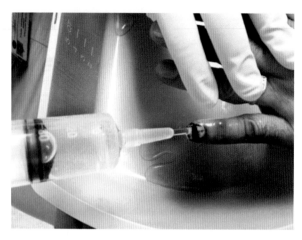

Fig. 10.5 Irrigating the nail bed for removal of hematoma or debris

- Debride the laceration edges removing any irregularities that may be present with the iris scissors to ensure a smooth repair without tension.
- Using the small tissue elevator, the edges of the nail bed laceration can be slightly undermined from the underlying periosteum, mobilizing this tissue for repair (Figs 10.6A and B).
- Repair the laceration using 6-0 absorbable monofilament sutures tied in simple fashion (Fig. 10.6C).

2-Octylcyanoacrylate Repair

- Once the laceration site has been irrigated, debrided and prepared, a single layer of 2-octylcyanoacrylate is applied to the laceration site.
- The edges of the laceration are held reapproximated manually as the tissue adhesive dries (approximately 60–90 seconds).
- Once the first layer is dry, a second layer is applied and allowed to dry completely.

Eponychial Interposition

- Following repair of the laceration, either the removed nail plate or a piece of foil from the suture packaging can be used as a stent underneath the eponychial fold to provide space for new nail

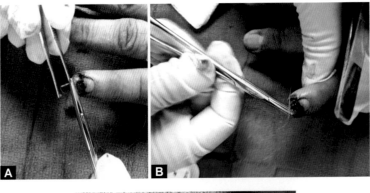

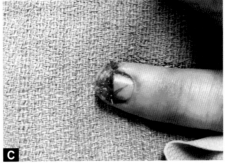

Figs 10.6A-C Repairing the laceration using 6-0 absorbable
monofilament sutures

growth and prevent the development of adhesions and later nail
plate deformity.
- This can trim/shape the edge of the removed nail plate ca be
  trimmed to easily fit underneath the eponychial fold.
- Either interposition choice can be held in place using either 6-0
  nylon suture or leftover 2-octylcyanoacrylate.
- For cases in which 6-0 nylon suture is used to hold the nail
  plate in place, the first pass is antegrade through the skin of the
  dorsum of the finger 5 mm proximal to the nail fold with the
  needle exiting between the eponychial fold and the nail bed.
  The next suture pass is through the prepared nail plate from
  posterior to anterior followed by another pass through the nail
  plate from anterior to posterior. The final suture pass is retro-
  grade starting between the eponychial fold and the nail bed

exiting through the skin of the dorsum of the finger approximately 5 mm proximal to the nail fold. Tension on the sutures will pull the nail plate into position underneath the eponychial fold. The sutures are then tied creating a horizontal mattress type configuration.

Dressings and Follow-up Care

- Xeroform, non-adherent gauze is then applied covering the nail bed repair.
- The finger is then wrapped in a kling dressing (Fig. 10.7).
- The repaired nail bed is then protected in a finger splint, immobilizing the DIP joint.
- Patients are discharged home with a 5-day course of oral antibiotics for prophylaxis against infection (cephalexin 250 mg PO qid)
- The repair site should be re-evaluated in 5 to 7 days.
- The interposed nail or suture packet foil can be removed from underneath the eponychial fold at three weeks post treatment.
- Educate the patient that new nail growth may take 3 to 6 months to occur and often some cosmetic deformity is present.

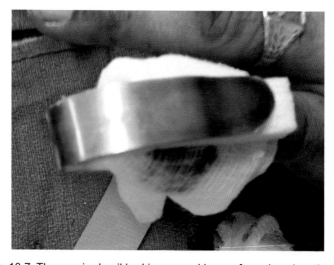

Fig. 10.7 The repaired nail bed is covered in xeroform dressing, the finger is wrapped in gauze and a splint is applied

SUGGESTED READINGS

1. Brown RE. Acute nail bed injuries. Hand Clin. 2002;18(4):561-75. Review

2. Elbeshbeshy BR, Rettig ME. Nail-bed repair and reconstruction. Tech Hand Up Extrem Surg. 2002;6(2):50-5. No abstract available.

3. Hart RG, Kleinert HE. Fingertip and nail bed injuries. Emerg Med Clin North Am. 1993;11(3):755-65. Review.

4. Strauss EJ, Weil WM, Jordan C, Paksima N. A prospective, randomized, controlled trial of 2-octylcyanoacrylate versus suture repair for nail bed injuries. J Hand Surg Am. 2008;33(2):250-3.

5. Van Beek AL, Kassan MA, Adson MH, Dale V. Management of acute fingernail injuries. Hand Clin. 1990;6(1):23-35; discussion 37-8. Review.

6. Zook EG, Guy RJ, Russell RC. A study of nail bed injuries: causes, treatment, and prognosis. J Hand Surg Am. 1984;9(2):247-52.

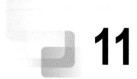

11

Closed Reduction of Pediatric Forearm Fractures

Eric J Strauss

INTRODUCTION

Forearm fractures in the pediatric patient population are very common injuries accounting for 45 percent of all fractures occurring in childhood and for 62 percent of fractures of the upper extremity.[4] Typically caused by falls at home or during athletic activities, 81 percent of pediatric forearm fractures occur in patients older than 5 years of age, with a peak incidence among boys 12 to 14 years old and girls 10 to 12 years old.[2,3] Reviews of pediatric forearm fractures have demonstrated that 75 to 84 percent occur in the distal third, 15–18 percent occur in the middle third and 1 to 7 percent occur in the proximal third.[1]

Fractures of the radius and ulna in children can be managed differently than those occurring in adults secondary to the continued growth and remodeling that occurs in the setting of open physes. Traditional treatment of pediatric forearm fractures includes closed reduction and cast immobilization. The following chapter will review the mechanisms of injury, methods of evaluation, classification and techniques for fracture reduction and casting.

MECHANISMS OF INJURY

Fractures of the pediatric radius and ulna may occur through either direct or indirect mechanisms. Direct injuries occur secondary to blunt trauma to the radius or ulnar shafts while the more common indirect injuries occur secondary to rotational mechanisms following a fall onto an outstretched hand. Pronation of the forearm during the fall typically results in a flexion type injury leading to dorsal angulation at the fracture site. Supination of the forearm during the fall leads to an extension type injury resulting in volar angulation at the fracture site.

PRESENTATION AND EVALUATION IN THE EMERGENCY ROOM

Patients with forearm fractures typically present to the emergency room (ER) with complaints of pain, swelling and difficulty with active use of the affected upper extremity. They may have gross deformity based on the extent of the injury.

The initial evaluation includes an inspection of the injured forearm, noting the presence of deformity and the condition of the surrounding soft tissue, looking for evidence of an open injury. A careful neurovascular examination should be performed and documented in the patient's chart. The location of forearm tenderness should be identified in addition to the presence of bony crepitus. Next, the ipsilateral hand, wrist and elbow should be palpated to rule out associated fractures or dislocations. In the case of dramatic forearm swelling, compartment syndrome should be ruled out based on serial neurovascular examinations and compartment pressure monitoring as indicated.

■ Radiographic Evaluation and Classification

Anteroposterior and lateral views of the forearm, wrist and elbow should be obtained in the evaluation of suspected pediatric forearm fractures (Fig. 11.1). This allows for characterization and classification of the forearm fracture in addition to ruling out associated injuries to the wrist (Galeazzi fracture) and elbow (Monteggia fracture or supracondylar humerus fracture).

Pediatric forearm fractures are classified according to the location of the injury, the type of fracture present and whether the fracture fragments are displaced or angulated. The location of the fracture is described as proximal, middle or distal third. Fracture types include plastic deformation (bending of the bone without fracture), compression or torus fractures (buckling of the bone), incomplete or

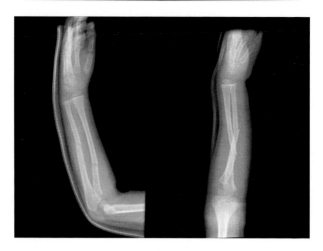

Fig. 11.1 Anteroposterior (AP) and lateral views of the forearm demonstrating a displaced both bones forearm fracture.

greenstick fractures (one cortex remains intact) and complete fractures occurring through both cortices.

Special fracture types occurring in the pediatric population include Galeazzi fractures in which a middle to distal third radius fracture occurs in the setting of an intact ulna with an associated disruption of the distal radioulnar joint. These fractures are relatively rare and typically present in patients having 9–12 years of age. Monteggia fractures are fractures of the proximal ulna occurring in association with a dislocation of the radial head. They are also rare injuries, typically occurring in patients 4–10 years of age.

REDUCTION OF PEDIATRIC FOREARM FRACTURES

The principles of management of pediatric forearm fractures include restoring anatomic alignment (both axial and rotational) and immobilizing in a well-molded long arm cast until fracture healing occurs. Understanding the deforming forces impacting the fracture fragments will make closed reduction of displaced forearm fractures easier (Fig. 11.2). In the proximal third of the radius, the supinator and biceps cause flexion and supination of the forearm. Inserting on the middle-third of the radius, the pronator teres causes pronation of the forearm. Distally, the pronator quadratus pronates the forearm.

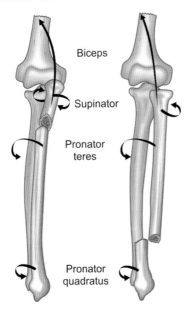

Biceps

Supinator

Pronator
teres

Pronator
quadratus

Fig. 11.2 Deforming forces in pediatric both bone forearm fractures (BBFAs).
Source: Adapted from Handbook of Fractures, 4th edition; 2010

Non-displaced fractures (torus fractures) or plastic deformation type injuries can be casted without manipulation until the fracture site is no longer tender to direct palpation. Greenstick and displaced fractures require manual manipulation to achieve anatomic reduction. The patient's age and fracture type will dictate whether the reduction can be performed under local anesthesia, conscious sedation or general anesthesia. A portable X-ray machine is recommended to check the quality of the reduction.

■ Technique

- Finger traps with or without weights on the upper arm can be used to facilitate the reduction maneuver (Fig. 11.3).
- Exaggeration of the deformity is necessary (often requiring more than 90°) to disengage the fracture fragments and associated periosteum, allowing for restoration of alignment and rotation.
- Once disengaged, the distal fragments can be apposed onto the end of the proximal fragments while simultaneously correcting the rotational alignment.

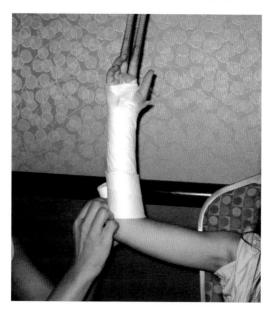

Fig. 11.3 Finger traps are used to help facilitate the reduction maneuver

- The reduction can be maintained with continuous manual pressure on the side of the intact periosteum (concave side of the injury).
- Check the adequacy of the reduction with anteroposterior and lateral fluoroscopy.

Cast Application

Following reduction of a displaced forearm fracture, a long-arm plaster or fiberglass cast is applied to immobilize the fracture site. This is typically performed using 3-inch plaster or fiberglass rolls but different sizes may be necessary depending on the patient's size. Based on the deforming muscle forces that impact the fracture fragments some authors recommend immobilizing proximal third forearm fractures in supination, middle third fractures in neutral and distal third fractures in pronation.

Materials Required

Materials required are rolls of plaster or fiberglass, a stockinette with a hole created for the thumb, rolls of cotton undercast padding, a basin of room temperature water and elastic bandages (used after the cast is bivalved).

- The patients' fingers are taken out of the finger traps allowing the stockinette to be applied to the upper extremity (Fig. 11.4). Once the stockinette is in place, the fingers can be re-hung to facilitate cast application.

  The elbow should be flexed to approximately 80° to avoid excessive pressure and compression at the elbow crease.

- To protect the underlying soft tissues, 2–3 layers of cotton undercast padding (webril) are applied, making sure no creases or folds are present as this will irritate the skin and can cause pressure injury under the splint (Fig. 11.5). Attention should be paid to the amount of undercast padding present in the elbow flexion crease to avoid unnecessary compression at this site.

- The first roll of plaster or fiberglass is applied, extending from the upper arm just distal to the axilla distally to the flexion

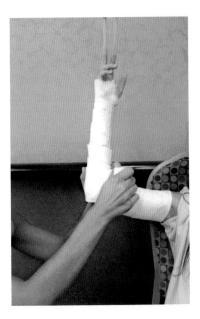

Fig. 11.4 Two to three layers of cotton undercast padding are applied to the patient's upper extremity. Care is taken to adequately pad the olecranon bony prominence

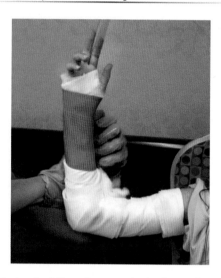

Fig. 11.5 The first roll of fiberglass or plaster is applied extending from the upper arm just distal to the axilla to the metacarpophalangeal (MCP) joints dorsally and the flexion crease of the palm volarly

crease of the palm (Figs 11.6A and B). The wrist should be in slight palmar-flexion and ulnar deviation. Care should be taken to avoid excess cast material around the thumb helping maintain flexion and extension at the thumb's metacarpophalangeal joint.

- Once the first layer of cast material has been applied, the ends of the stockinette can be folded over the edges of the cast.
- The second layer of plaster or fiberglass is then applied as shown in Figure 11.7 (if plaster is used as the cast material additional layers may be necessary to provide stability).
- As the cast material is hardening, a firm interosseous mold is applied to the fracture site (Figs 11.8A and B), maintaining pressure both volarly and dorsally.
7. If swelling is a concern, the cast can be bivalved with a cast saw and overwrapped with an elastic bandage (Figs 11.9A and B).

An additional layer of cast material will be applied in the office at the first follow up visit once the injury-associated swelling has subsided.

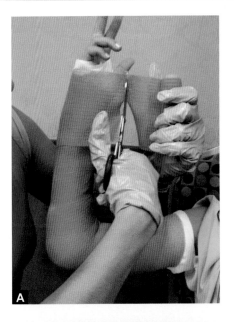

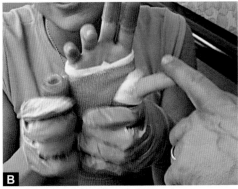

Figs 11.6A and B In the region of the palm the fiberglass is cut to facilitate wrapping around the thumb, leaving room for free motion at the thumb metacarpophalangeal (MCP) joint

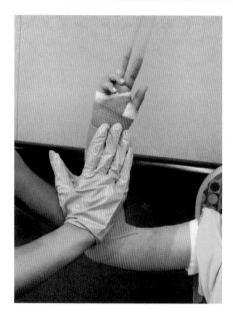

Fig. 11.7 A firm interosseous mold is applied with the physician's palms

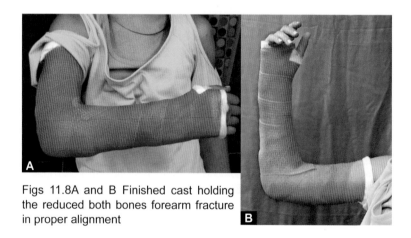

Figs 11.8A and B Finished cast holding the reduced both bones forearm fracture in proper alignment

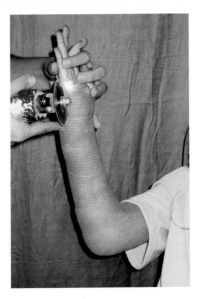

Figs 11.9 The cast is bivalved using a cast saw to allow for post-injury swelling to occur without complication. The bivalved cast is overwrapped with an elastic bandage

POST-REDUCTION CARE

Once the cast has hardened, the patient should be sent for a repeat forearm X-ray series to confirm adequate fracture reduction (Figs 11.10A and B). Once an acceptable reduction is confirmed the patient is placed in a sling for comfort. The patient is followed with weekly X-rays for the first three weeks to check for any fracture site displacement. Re-displacement has been noted to occur in up to 13 percent of cases, typically occurring within two weeks of the injury.[1,4] Pediatric forearm fractures typically require 4–6 weeks of cast immobilization for healing to occur. If healing is found to be progressing at 3 to 4 weeks, the patient may be converted to a short arm cast at that time.

Emergency Room Orthopaedic Procedures

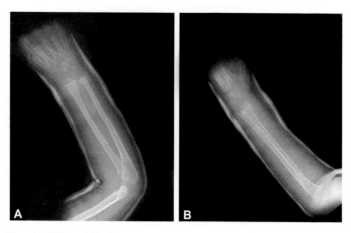

Figs 11.10A and B   Post-reduction anteroposterior (AP) and lateral
X-ray views confirming adequate fracture reduction

REFERENCES

1. Armstrong PF, Clarke HM. Pediatric fractures of the forearm, wrist and
    hand. Skeletal Trauma in Children. Philadelphia: Saunders; 1998. pp.
    161-257.
2. Bailey DA, Wedge JH, McCulloch RG, et al. Epidemiology of fractures
    of the distal end of the radius in children as associated with growth. J
    Bone Joint Surg Am. 1989;71(8): 1225-31.
3. Kramhoft M, Bodtker S. Epidemiology of distal forearm fractures in
    Danish children. Acta Orthop Scand. 1988;59(5):557-9.
4. Rodriguez-Merchan EC. Pediatric fractures of the forearm. Clin Orthop
    Relat Res. 2005;(432):65-72.

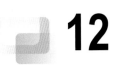

12

Diagnosis of Compartment Syndrome

Kenneth A Egol

INTRODUCTION

Compartment syndrome is a condition characterized by elevated pressure within a closed space such that tissue oxygenation is compromised. It has the potential to cause irreversible damage to the contents of that closed space. This is a limb-threatening condition with several severe long-term consequences, if left untreated. Many of the late sequelae associated with compartment syndrome can be avoided by early diagnosis and treatment.

PATHOPHYSIOLOGY

Compartment syndrome can be due to either an increase in the contents of the compartment or a decreased volume within a compartment. Situations that cause an increased volume include hemorrhage, fracture, increased fluid secondary to burns and post-ischemic swelling. The most common cause of decreased volume is a tight cast. Most common anatomic locations for compartment syndrome include the leg, elbow, forearm and thigh. Muscle injury secondary to trauma leads to edema. The presence of a fracture exacerbates this situation secondary to fracture hematoma; this further increases the volume within the compartment. Ischemia-reperfusion injury on a cellular level involves damage to the cellular basement membrane that results in edema. With re-establishment of flow, fluid leaks into the compartment increasing its volume. A continuous increase in pressure within a compartment occurs until the low intramuscular arteriolar pressure is exceeded and blood cannot enter the capillaries. If no further blood enters the compartment and shunting occurs, nerve and muscle ischemia soon follows. Muscle can survive up to 4 hours without irreversible damage. A total ischemia of greater than 8 hours produces complete and irreversible changes in muscle. By 4 hours of ischemia, neuropraxia is irreversible. Axonotmesis and irreversible changes occur in nerves after 8 hours of total ischemia time.

PERTINENT ANATOMY

■ Leg

The anterior, lateral and superficial posterior compartments of the leg are all subcutaneous; therefore their pressures can be measured directly. The anterior compartment contains the tibialis anterior, extensor digitorum longus, the extensor hallucis longus and the peroneus tertius muscles. The lateral compartment contains the peroneus longus and brevis muscles. The superficial posterior compartment contains the gastrocnemius and soleus muscles. The deep posterior compartment contains the tibialis posterior, the flexor hallucis longus and the flexor digitorum muscles. Distally, the deep posterior compartment is subcutaneous and its pressures can be measured medial and posterior to the tibia.

■ Thigh

There are three compartments in the thigh. These include the anterior compartment, which contains the quadriceps group; the posterior compartment which contains the hamstring muscles and; the medial compartment containing the adductor muscle group. A thick intermuscular septum separates the three compartments.

■ Forearm

The forearm can be divided into three compartments: dorsal, volar and "mobile wad". The mobile wad contains the brachioradialis, extensor carpi radialis longus (ECRL), extensor carpi radialis brevis (ECRB). The dorsal compartment of the forearm contains the extensor pollicis brevis (EPB), extensor pollicis longus (EPL), extensor carpi ulnaris (ECU), extensor digitorum communis (EDC). The volar forearm compartment contains flexor pollicis longus (FPL), flexor carpi radialis (FCR), flexor carpi ulnaris (FCU), flexor digitorum superficialis (FDS), flexor digitorum profundus (FDP), palmaris longus (PL).

■ Arm

The arm includes the anterior and posterior compartments, divided by the intermuscular septum. The anterior compartment contains the biceps, brachialis and coracobrachialis. The posterior compartment contains three heads of the triceps and the anconeus.

In the leg, compartment syndromes are most common in the deep posterior and the anterior compartments. In the forearm, they occur most frequently in the volar compartment, especially in the deep flexor area.

DIAGNOSIS

The clinical findings in a patient with compartment syndrome are often not clear cut. A tense, swollen compartment is not always obvious, especially if there is only involvement of the deep posterior compartment of leg. The classic signs of the "5 P's": pain, pallor, paralysis, pulselessness and paresthesias are not always reliable. These are signs of an established compartment syndrome where ischemic injury has already taken place. Palpable pulses are usually present in acute compartment syndromes unless an arterial injury occurs. Paralysis and sensory changes do not occur until ischemia has been present for about one hour or more. The most important symptom of an impending compartment syndrome is pain out of proportion to what would be expected. Pain on passive stretch of muscles within the compartment is also a sensitive sign. These signs are only useful in responsive patients. Pain becomes less reliable after muscle necrosis and nerve ischemia has occurred. The presence of an open fracture does not rule out the presence of a compartment syndrome. Many open tibial fractures are associated with compartment syndromes. McQueen et al found no significant differences in compartment pressures between open and closed tibial fractures.

Also, they found no significant difference in pressures between tibial fractures treated with intramedullary nails and those treated with external fixation.

As clinical signs are not always obvious and may be masked by the patient's associated injuries or mental status, tissue pressure measurements are often utilized. There has been disagreement over what pressure values are indicative of compartment syndrome. Early thought supported fasciotomies for tissue-pressures greater than 30 mm Hg. Matsen et al suggested fasciotomies for pressures more than 45 mm Hg. Whitesides et al in 1975 was the first to suggest that the significance of tissue, pressures was in their relation to diastolic blood pressure. He recommended fasciotomies for tissue, pressures within 10–30 mm Hg of the diastolic pressure. In their prospective study of 116 patients with closed diaphyseal tibial fractures, McQueen et al. found that absolute compartment pressure is an unreliable indication for the need for fasciotomies. They concluded that fasciotomy is indicated when the difference between the compartment pressure and diastolic blood pressure is less than 30 mm Hg. Thus, in hypotensive and hypertensive patients, the absolute pressure causing a compartment syndrome will be lower and higher, respectively. Using this guideline, no compartment syndromes were missed. Heckman et al demonstrated that pressure within a given compartment is not uniform. They found tissue pressures to be highest at the site or within 5 cm of the injury, with clinically and statistically significant changes in pressure occurring at distances as little as 5 cm from the site of highest pressure. Three of their five patients requiring fasciotomies had sub-critical pressure values 5 cm from the site of highest pressure. Simple palpation of the extremity to determine the site at which to perform the measurement cannot guarantee that the area of highest pressure is being measured. Therefore, when measuring compartment pressures, multiple measurements should be taken in order to assure the site of maximal pressure has been measured. Measurements should be taken at the level of the fracture and at locations both proximal and distal to the fracture. Multiple techniques exist for measuring tissue pressures: needle manometer, wick catheter, slit catheter and stic catheter. Moed et al demonstrated that the slit catheter and side-ported needle are equally accurate and that the simple needle technique obtained higher pressure values should not be used.

The needle-infusion technique can be done with basic hospital equipment. In this technique, a 20 ml syringe is attached to three-way stopcock; one end connected to manometer, the other end to an extension tube half-filled with saline. The stopcock is open to both extensions. The needle is inserted into muscle and the tube with saline kept at this height. If the pressure in tissue is greater than air column, saline forms convex meniscus away from patient. As plunger is depressed, the meniscus changes from convex to flat and at this level, it is equivalent to tissue pressure. Increased pressure causes a concave meniscus.

A battery powered compartment pressure monitor (Stryker) can be utilized in the acute setting with very reliable results. This device involves a saline filled tube and syringe attached to a pressure gauge and needle. The technique is similar to that of Whitesides without the need for a complicated set up.

Leg Compartment Measurement Technique (Using Stryker Compartment Pressure Monitor)

All four compartments should be measured: the anterior, lateral, superficial posterior and deep posterior compartments. The anterior and lateral compartments are usually measured from the lateral side of the leg. The posterior compartments are usually measured from the medial side of the leg. If a fracture is present, the measurement should be made as close to the level of the fracture.

The lateral compartment is measured in line with the fibula or posterior to it (Fig. 12.1). The anterior compartment is measured over the muscle belly between the fibula and the anterior crest of the tibia.

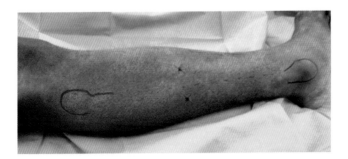

Fig. 12.1 The anatomic landmarks of the lateral aspect of the lower leg are marked out including the outline of the fibula

The superficial posterior compartment is measured over the posteromedial aspect of the gastrocsoleus complex.

The deep posterior compartment is measured in the distal one half of the leg along the posteromedial border of the tibia. This compartment is the most difficult to measure accurately.

The Stryker compartment pressure monitor is assembled as shown in Figure 12.2.

The unit is turned on and should read between 0 mm Hg and 9 mm Hg. The trocar needle is placed on the tapered chamber stem and the cap is removed from the pre-filled syringe. The syringe is screwed on to the remaining chamber stem. One must take care not to contaminate the fluid pathway. The cover of the monitor is opened and chamber is placed in the round well (black surface down) and pushed until seated. The cover of the monitor is closed. The syringe cap is then removed and the plunger attached. Holding the needle at 45° up from horizontal, fluid is lowly forced through the syringe and needle to eliminate air within the system.

Once the correct needle placement locations are determined, the skin is prepped with an antiseptic solution. The Stryker compartment pressure monitor is then zeroed at the level of the intended measurement location by pressing the zero button and waiting for the display to read "00". The needle is inserted through the skin and into the intended compartment. Less than 0.3 cc of fluid is injected into the compartment to equilibrate with the interstitial fluids. One must

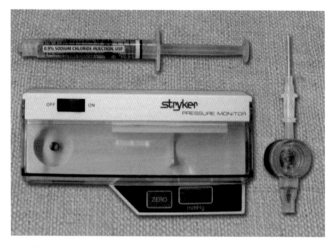

Fig. 12.2 The Stryker compartment pressure monitor

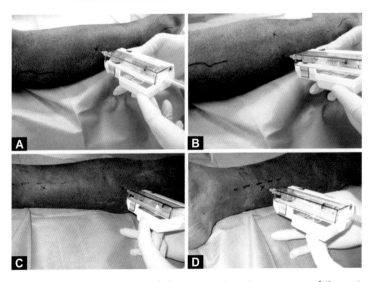

Figs 12.3A-D Measurement of the compartment pressures of the anterior compartment (A) lateral compartment (B) superficial posterior compartment (C) and the deep posterior compartment (D) using the Stryker compartment pressure monitor. A distal line demarcating the posterior edge of the tibia is used as a reference to confirm needle placement within the deep posterior compartment

wait for the display to reach equilibrium and the pressure recorded (Figs 12.3A-D). These steps are repeated at each additional pressure measurement site.

Leg Compartment Pressure Measurement Technique (Needle Infusion Technique)

If a battery powered compartment pressure monitor is not available for use, a system can be set up using available hospital equipment. Supplies include a 20 ml syringe attached to three-way stopcock with one end connected to manometer and the other end to an extension tube half-filled with saline. The stopcock is open to both extensions. The needle is inserted into the compartment in the same manner as described above and the tube with saline kept at this height. If the pressure in tissue is greater than air column, the saline forms convex meniscus away from patient. As plunger is depressed forcing fluid into the tissue, meniscus changes from convex to flat.

At this level, the measured pressure is equivalent to tissue pressure. Increased pressure causes a change in the meniscus to concave away from the patient.

SUGGESTED READINGS

1. Allen MJ, Stirling AJ, Crawshaw CV, et al. Intracompartmental pressure monitoring of leg injuries: An aid to management. J Bone Joint Surg Br. 1985;67B:53-7.

2. Amendola A, Twaddle BC. Compartment syndromes. In: Browner BD, Jupiter JB, Levine AM, Trafton PG (Eds). Skeletal Trauma, Vol. 1, 2nd edition. Philadelphia: WB Saunders Company; 1998. pp. 365-89.

3. Azar FM. Traumatic disorders. In: Canale TS (Ed). Campbell's Operative Orthopaedics, 10th edition. Philadelphia: Mosby; 2003. pp. 2449-93.

4. Gelberman RH, Szabo RM, Williamson RV, et al. Tissue pressure threshold for peripheral nerve viability. Clin Orthop Relat Res. 1983;(178):285-91.

5. Kahan JSG, McClellan RT, Burton DS. Acute bilateral compartment syndrome of the thigh induced by exercise. J Bone Joint Surg Am. 1994;76:1068-71.

6. Kuklo TR, Tis JE, Moores LK, et al. Fatal rhabdomyolysis with bilateral gluteal, thigh, and leg compartment syndrome after the army physical fitness test. A case report. Am J Sports Med. 2000;28:112-6.

7. Matsen FA, Winquist RA, Krugmire RB. Diagnosis and management of compartmental syndromes. J Bone Joint Surg Am. 1980;62A:286-91.

8. Mubarak SJ, Owen CA, Hargens AR, et al. Acute compartment syndromes: diagnosis and treatment with the aid of the wick catheter. J Bone Joint Surg Am. 1978;60:1091-5.

9. Nau T, Menth-Chiari WA, Seitz H, et al. Acute compartment syndrome of the thigh associated with exercise. Am J Sports Med. 2000;28:120-2.

10. Schwartz JT, Brumback RJ, Lakatos R, et al. Acute compartment syndrome of the thigh. A spectrum of injury. J Bone Joint Surg Am. 1989;71:392-9.

11. Tarlow SD, Achterman CA, Hayhurst J, et al. Acute compartment syndrome in the thigh complicating fracture of the femur. A sreport of three cases. J Bone Joint Surg Am. 1986;68:1439-43.

12. Viegas SF, Rimoldi R, Scarborough M, et al. Acute compartment syndrome in the thigh. A case report and review of the literature. Clin Orthop Relat Res. 1988;234:232-4.

13. Whitesides TE, Haney TC, Morimoto K, et al. Tissue pressure measurements as a determinant for the need of fasciotomy. Clin Orthop Relat Res. 1975;113:43-51.

13

Suturing Lacerations in the Emergency Room

Sonya Khurana, Eric J Strauss

INTRODUCTION

Laceration repair is a common procedure performed in the emergency room. Fifty percent of lacerations occur on the head or neck and 35 percent occur on the upper extremity, especially the fingers or hands. Goals of repair include hemostasis, restoration of function, cosmesis and prevention of infection.

When a patient presents to the emergency department with a laceration, the wound should be evaluated under proper lighting for the severity of injury (involvement of muscles, tendons, bone, nerves and blood vessels), bleeding and the presence of any foreign bodies or devitalized tissue. Bleeding should be controlled using direct pressure and/or epinephrine (epinephrine should not be used in areas with end arterioles, such as the digit, nose, penis and earlobes). If an extremity is involved, a tourniquet may be utilized. Foreign bodies should be removed with forceps and devitalized tissue should be sharply debrided. A neurovascular exam should be performed prior to anesthesia. The wound should be irrigated with warmed normal saline. Antibiotics may be necessary depending upon the level of contamination and tissue devitalization. The patient's tetanus immunization history should be obtained.

Non-contaminated wounds should be closed within 12 hours of injury or may be packed for 3 to 5 days with delayed primary closure following. Extremity lacerations should be repaired within 19 hours so that healing is not impaired. If the wound is infected, it should left to heal by secondary intention. Clipping hair around the area can also help prevent infection.

ANESTHESIA

It is necessary to anesthetize the area around the laceration for the patient's comfort during laceration repair. Small wounds can be locally anesthetized with lidocaine 1 percent or bupivacaine 0.25 percent. In patients who are allergic to these agents, diphenhydramine diluted to 1 percent can be used. The injection can be made less painful by using a smaller gauge needle (25 to 30 gauge), injecting slowly, warming the anesthetic or buffering the solution with sodium bicarbonate. Topical anesthetics like eutectic mixture of local anesthetics (EMLA) can also be used and are especially helpful in children. They should be applied 1 to 4 hours before laceration repair. Large wounds on limbs may require a regional block.

Although there is a few ways of repairing lacerations, such as suturing, use of tissue adhesives, skin closure tape and staples. This chapter will focus on suturing, as it is still the most common method of laceration repair.

SUPPLIES

Sutures are especially important in repairing lacerations in high tension areas like joints or areas with a thick dermis, such as the back. Absorbable sutures are used to close deep, multilayer lacerations and include Vicryl (Ethicon Inc., Somerville NJ), Dexon (Covididen, Dublin, Ireland), and Monocryl (Ethicon Inc, Somerville NJ). These sutures absorb within four to eight weeks. Nonabsorbable sutures include prolene and nylon, and they must be removed. The sutures are fairly nonreactive and can hold their tensile strength for more than 60 days. Synthetic and monofilament sutures have decreased rates of infection compared with natural (i.e. catgut) and braided sutures. The finest suture possible should be used for optimal cosmetic results. A 3-0 or 4-0 suture is usually used on the trunk and a 4-0 or 5-0 suture is used on the extremities and visible scalp. The deep, multilayer wounds should be repaired with single interrupted, absorbable sutures. Other wounds can be repaired with nonabsorbable, single interrupted sutures. The suture starts in the middle of the wound for large wounds, with the rest of the stitches places symmetrically in a lateral fashion.

There are many different ways to suture and their use depends on the characteristics of the wound. Horizontal mattress sutures spread the tension along the wound edge and are therefore, beneficial for closing gaping or high-tension wounds or wounds on fragile skin. The vertical mattress sutures are best for everting wound edges in areas that tend to invert, such as the posterior neck or concave skin surfaces. A running "baseball" suture is used for long, low-tension wounds. A subcuticular running stitch is ideal for small lacerations in low skin-tension areas where cosmesis is important, such as on the face.

Instruct patients to keep the wound clean and dry for at least 24 to 48 hours. This allows enough epithelialization to occur to protect the wound from gross contamination. They can also apply antibiotic or white petrolatum ointment daily to the wound to prevent infection and promote healing. Sutures on the forearm can be removed in 10 to 14 days, those on the fingers and hand in 8 to 10 days, those in the lower extremity at 8 to 12 days and those in the foot at 10 to 12 days. Sutures in high tension areas such as the joints and hands should be left in for 10 to 14 days.

MATERIALS

Materials required are normal saline, sterile needle driver, Adson forceps, sterile suture material on needle (see previously in the chapter for type of suture needed), local anesthetic, sterile scissors, alcohol wipes and gloves.

STEPS

■ Simple Interrupted Stitch

- Irrigate the laceration with normal saline and remove any foreign bodies.
- Prepare the skin around the laceration with an alcohol wipe or Betadine and inject local anesthetic around the wound, such as 1 percent lidocaine buffered in a 1:10 ratio with sodium bicarbonate 8.4 percent.
- Place the needle in the tip of the needle driver, about 60 percent back from the pointed end of the needle.
- Using the Adson forceps, grasp and slightly evert the skin edge of one end of the wound.

- Hold the hand with the needle driver in pronation, with the needle positioned to pierce the skin at a 90° angle.
- Pierce the skin with the needle and supinate the hand holding the needle driver in order to bring the needle through the first skin edge.
- Release the needle from the needle holder and pronate the hand. Re-grasp the needle with the needle driver.
- Grasp the second skin edge with the forceps and evert it slightly.
- Supinate the hand in order to rotate the needle through the skin.
- Release the needle, pronate the hand and re-grasp the needle.
- Supinate the hand to bring the remainder of the needle through the skin. Leave approximately 2 to 4 cm of suture material hanging from the first skin edge.
- Place the needle driver between the two suture strands and over the wound. Set down or palm the forceps.
- Wrap the long end of the suture around the needle driver twice in order to throw a square knot.
- Grasp the short end of the suture with the needle driver and bring it back through the loop. Tighten the throw and make sure that it lies flat on the skin.
- Repeat steps 13 and 14 about three times, but wrap the long end of the suture around the needle driver only once each time.
- Cut the suture and leave a 3 mm tail. Place the next stitch about 3 to 4 mm away from the first one, though this will vary depending on how easily the wound edges can be approximated. A laceration on a flexion surface usually requires closer sutures.
- After the repair is complete, clean the wound with sterile saline and dress it. Lacerations over joints may be splinted temporarily for comfort and to promote healing.

■ Simple Running Suture

- Follow steps 1 to 15 described above for the simple interrupted technique. Do not cut the suture after step 15.
- Start the next stitch about 3 to 4 mm away from the first one and repeat steps 4 to 11 as outlined above. Do not tie any knots or cut any suture.
- Repeat the above step until the entire length of the wound is closed (Figs 13.1A and B).
- Wrap the long end of the suture around the needle driver twice

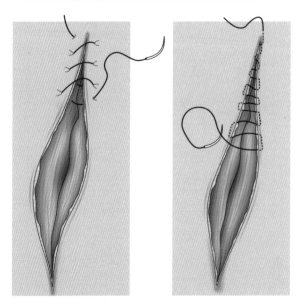

Figs 13.1A and B For subcuticular closure, needle passes are made deep to the surface at the junction of the epidermis and dermis. (A) Schematic of a simple running suture; (B) Running subcuticular suture

and grab the same end of the suture with the needle driver in order to throw a square knot (Fig. 13.2).

- Cut the suture and leave a 3 mm tail.
- After the repair is complete, clean the wound with sterile saline and dress it. Lacerations over joints may be splinted temporarily for comfort and to promote healing.

■ Vertical Mattress Suture

- Irrigate the laceration with normal saline and remove any foreign bodies.
- Prep the skin around the laceration with an alcohol wipe and inject local anesthetic around the wound.
- Place the needle in the tip of the needle driver, about 60 percent back from the pointed end of the needle.
- Hold the hand with the needle driver in pronation, with the needle positioned to pierce the skin at a 90° angle about 4 to 8 mm from the wound edge.

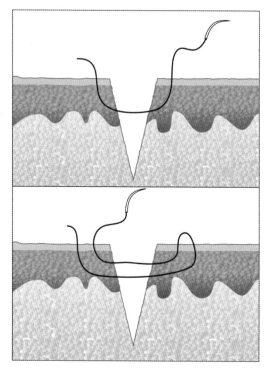

Fig. 13.2 Schematic of a vertical mattress suture

- Pierce the skin deep below the dermis.
- Pass the needle through the inside of the second skin edge and supinate the hand as the needle is brought through the skin. Leave a 3 to 4 cm tail of suture.
- Place the needle backwards in the needle driver and position it about 5 mm from where the needle came out of the skin.
- Pierce the skin at a shallow depth in the upper dermis and 1 to 2 mm away from the wound edge. Pass the needle through the near edge of the skin and across the wound through the far edge of the skin.
- Place the needle driver between the two suture strands.
- Wrap the long end of the suture around the needle driver twice in order to throw a square knot (Fig. 13.2). The knot should be on the side where the suture passage began.

- Grasp the short end of the suture with the needle driver and bring it back through the loop. Tighten the throw and make sure it lies flat on the skin.
- Repeat steps 13 and 14 about three times, but wrap the long end of the suture around the needle driver only once each time.
- Cut the suture and leave a 3 mm tail. Place the next stitch about 3 to 4 mm away from the first one, though this will vary depending on how easily the wound edges can be approximated. A laceration on a flexion surface usually requires closer sutures.
- After the repair is complete, clean the wound with sterile saline and dress it. Lacerations over joints may be splinted temporarily for comfort and to promote healing.

SUGGESTED READINGS

1. Berk WA, Osbourne DD, Taylor DD. Evaluation of the "golden period" for wound repair: 204 cases from a third world emergency department. Ann Emerg Med. 1988;17:496-500.
2. Capellan O, Hollander JE. Management of lacerations in the emergency department. Emerg Med Clin North Am. 2003;21:205-31.
3. Forsch RT. Essentials of skin laceration repair. Am Fam Physician. 2008;78(8):945-51.
4. Singer AJ, Hollander JE, Quinn JV. Evaluation and management of traumatic lacerations. New England Journal of Medicine. 1997;337(16):1142-8.
5. Zuber TJ. The mattress sutures: Vertical, horizontal, and corner stitch. Am Fam Physician. 2002;66(12):2231-6.

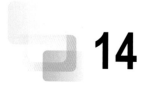

14

Pediatric and Adult Procedural Sedation and Analgesia

Robert C Rothberg

PROCEDURAL SEDATION AND ANALGESIA

Procedural sedation and analgesia (PSA) is a technique of administering sedatives or dissociative agents with or without analgesics to induce a state that allows the patient to tolerate unpleasant procedures while maintaining cardiopulmonary function. This technique is characterized by a drug-induced state of depressed consciousness that permits preservation of protective airway reflexes, maintenance of a patent airway by the patient and their ability to respond appropriately to verbal or tactile stimulus. It is important that the provider recognizes that sedation is a continuum from minimal sedation through moderate sedation (formally referred to as conscious sedation) and deep sedation to general anesthesia. These discrete levels of consciousness on the continuum of sedation are not well defined and the interobserver variability is high in judging the depth of sedation for an individual patient. Additionally, since it is difficult to predict the response of any given patient to a particular procedural sedation agent, the clinician administering the medication needs to possess the skill set necessary to deal with a depth of sedation deeper than intended, including advanced airway and critical care skills. Most procedural sedation agents used in the emergency setting have a dose-response relationship, including benzodiazepines (i.e. midazolam), opioids (i.e. morphine, fentanyl), propofol, etomidate. Ketamine is an exception and is discussed here.

■ Requirements Prior to Procedural Sedation

Prior to procedural sedation, a complete patient assessment is required. Pertinent aspects of the patient history include identifying allergies or previous reactions to particular procedural sedation agents, comorbidities to detect possible contraindications to particular procedural sedation agents [i.e. snoring/sleep apnea, congestive heart failure, advanced rheumatoid arthritis (especially of cervical spine)]. An assessment of the patient's overall health is mandatory, typically using the ASA classification system (Table 14.1).

An assessment of the patients' fasting state is also important with respect to the time of their last solid food or liquid ingestion. At the present time, there is a lack of evidence that gastric emptying has any impact on the incidence of complications or on outcome in procedural sedation and analgesia. According to the current American College of Emergency Physicians (ACEPs) clinical policy guidelines, recent food intake is not a contraindication for administering procedural sedation and analgesia, but should be considered in choosing the timing and level of sedation. The American Society of Anesthesiologists (ASA) has provided guidelines for pre-procedure fasting that should be considered for patients requiring procedural sedation and anesthesia (Table 14.2).

The physical examination of patients prior to procedural sedation and anesthesia should assess for anticipated airway management issues, including any craniofacial abnormalities, the status of the neck and cervical range of motion, the appearance of the mouth and jaw and whether or not any loose teeth are present. The heart

Table 14.1	ASA classification
Class 1	Healthy
Class 2	Mild systemic disease
Class 3	Severe but not incapacitating systemic disease
Class 4	Incapacitating systemic disease that is constant threat to life
Class 5	Moribund patient not likely to survive more than 24 hours

Note: In general, PSA should be limited to patients in class 1 and 2. Consultation with anesthesiologist is recommended for patients of class 4 and above.

Table 14.2	ASA Pre-procedure Fasting Guidelines
Ingested food	*Minimum fasting period recommended*
Clear liquids	2 hours
Breast milk	4 hours
Infant formula	6 hours
Non-human milk	6 hours
Light meal	6 hours

and lungs should be assessed for evidence of active bronchospasm or congestive heart failure.

An upper airway assessment can be performed according to the modified Mallampati classification, based on the degree of visualization of the uvula, soft palate and faucial pillars when the patient is asked to maximally open their mouth from a sitting position.

According to this classification, Class 0 describes the ability to visualize all three structures and epiglottis. Class 1 describes the ability to visualize all three structures (as well as hard palate). In Class 2 upper airway, the examiner can only visualize the uvula and soft palate. In Class 3, the examiner can only visualize base of uvula and soft palate and in Class 4, the examiner can only visualize the hard palate. According to this classification system patients with Class 3 and 4 upper airways are associated with higher rates of intubation difficulty and failure should securing an airway become necessary during sedation.

Prior to the start of procedural sedation and anesthesia, signed informed consent for both the procedural sedation and the associated procedure should be obtained.

Necessary Supplies for Procedural Sedation and Anesthesia

For procedural sedation and anesthesia, intravenous access, the appropriate agents, tools and staff for continuous patient monitoring, all are required in addition to age-appropriate resuscitation equipment (with reversal agents if opioids or benzodiazepines are being administered). The monitoring individual should be a clinician (RN or MD) with advanced airway skills (ACLS/PALS) who is exclusively assigned to observe the patient and their clinical parameters during the procedure. Required supplies include a cardiac monitor for monitoring blood pressure, heart rate, respiratory rate and O_2 saturation.

Whether or not capnometry (continuous end-tidal CO_2 monitoring) is indicated for procedural sedation and anesthesia is a subject of debate. Advantages include that it is noninvasive, simple to apply, monitor and interpret in addition to provide the earliest indication of respiratory depression (hypoventilation) and thus hypoxia, even before this, is reflected by a decreased oxygen saturation. Cited disadvantages include the fact that most episodes of hypoxemia are transient, do not require intervention and frequently not clinically significant. Additionally, respiratory depression is usually clinically apparent and quickly reflected in oxygen saturation, therefore the slightly earlier warning provided by capnometry is of questionable additional benefit coming at the expense of another parameter that requires continuous monitoring. Our recommendation is to consider monitoring end-tidal CO_2 in situations where respiratory depression is likely to result (use of propofol) or where a patient would poorly tolerate even a brief period of hypoxemia.

■ Techniques for Procedural Sedation and Anesthesia

- Pre-procedure time out confirming the correct patient, procedure, laterality or level.
- Administration of supplemental oxygen: This is also a subject of debate. Cited advantages include the belief that a pre-oxygenated patient has a higher oxygen reserve so that he can tolerate a longer period of respiratory depression or apnea before becoming hypoxemic. Disadvantages include the fact that supplemental oxygen may mask and delay the recognition of respiratory depression by pulse oximetry. Using supplemental oxygen is recommended in situations where respiratory depression is likely to result (use of propofol) or where a patient would poorly tolerate even a brief period of hypoxemia. The use of supplemental oxygen is documented just prior to start of procedural sedation, every 5 minutes during sedation, then every 10 minutes during recovery phase until return to pre-sedation baseline.

- Administration of the sedation/anesthesia agents: Specific agents used for procedural sedation and anesthesia discussed below.
- Assessment of mental status and the depth of sedation: It can be classified according to the Ramsay Sedation Score.
  - 1 point: Anxious and agitated or restless, or both
  - 2 points: Cooperative, oriented and tranquil
  - 3 points: Responds to commands only
  - 4 points: Brisk response to light glabellar tap or loud auditory stimulus
  - 5 points: Sluggish response to light glabellar tap or loud auditory stimulus
  - 6 points: No response
- Continuous monitoring of vital signs by monitoring clinician including blood pressure, heart rate, oxygen saturation +/− endtidal CO_2.
- Determination of discharge criteria (discussed below).

Choosing the Appropriate Procedural Sedation Agent

The providing clinician should determine the category of the underlying procedure for which procedural sedation is needed (Table 14.3). This includes reduction of orthopedic fractures or dislocations, reduction, laceration repair, incision and drainage of an abscess, foreign body removal or an imaging procedure. The provider must ask what characteristics will be required for sedation including analgesia for painful procedures, sedation for anxiolysis, and cooperation and amnesia for the procedure, the anticipated duration of the procedure requiring sedation and the general health and comorbidities of the patient in order to determine contraindications for particular agents.

▌Discharge Criteria Following Procedural Sedation and Anesthesia

Guidelines for discharge following procedural sedation and anesthesia have been developed. Patients must be alert and oriented and back to their pre-sedation baseline with stable vital signs. Their neurologic examination should be back to their baseline with respect to their motor, sensory and cerebellar function. If patient was capable of walking in, they should be able to walk out (perhaps with minimal assistance if minimal ataxia persists from sedation agent). If reversal

Table 14.3 Procedural sedation agents

Agent	Indication	Dosing	Adverse effects	Summary
Etomidate	For use in both pediatric and adult patients. May need to administer a concomitant analgesic for a painful procedure	Initial bolus of 0.1 mg/kg IV Additional dosing: 0.05 mg/kg IV every 3–5 minutes	Nausea/vomiting, respiratory depression, myoclonus and post-sedation myalgias, injection site pain	Ultrashort-acting sedative-hypnotic agent with an onset of action of 30–60 seconds and duration of action from 5–15 minutes. Etomidate possesses sedative and amnestic properties but does not possess analgesic properties
Propofol	For use in both adult and pediatric patients May need to administer an analgesic for a painful procedure	Initial bolus of 1 mg/kg followed by 0.5 mg/kg every 3 minutes titrated to achieve/maintain desired level of sedation Recommend maximum initial dose of 40 mg in pediatric patients Alternate protocol for adult patients: Mini boluses of 10–40 mg IV every 10–15 seconds titrated to the desired level of sedation, followed by 20 mg aliquots to maintain sedation	Respiratory depression, transient hypotension, injection site pain	Ultra-short acting non-opioid, non-barbiturate sedative-hypnotic agent with an onset of action of 30 seconds, duration of action of 6 minutes and recovery of time of approximately 10–30 minutes Propofol possesses sedative and hypnotic properties but does not possess analgesic properties

Contd...

Contd...

Versed-fentanyl combination	For procedural sedation in adults and pediatrics. However, this combination has become an increasingly second line option	**Adult:** Midazolam 0.02 mg/kg (maximum 2 mg), observe for 2–3 minutes, (may give additional midazolam until desired sedation reached, wait 2–3 minutes), then fentanyl 0.5 µg/kg, observe for 2–3 minutes, then titrate each drug to desired level of sedation/analgesia **Pediatric patients:** Midazolam initial dose: less than 0.1 mg/kg (maximum 2.5 mg) every 3 minutes until adequate sedation has occurred or total dose of 0.3 mg/kg (maximum 7.5 mg) given Wait 2–3 minutes after last dose of midazolam given, then fentanyl	Respiratory depression, hypotension, rigid chest wall syndrome (fentanyl)	This technique combines a short-acting benzodiazepine with synthetic opioid. Combined these agents have sedative, amnestic and analgesic properties Onset of action: Fentanyl: 2–3 minutes; versed: 2–5 minutes Duration of action: Fentanyl: 20–30 minutes; versed: 30–60 minutes

Contd...

Contd...

	less than 0.5 µg/kg is given every 3 minutes until adequate sedation/analgesia has occurred or total dose of 2 µg/kg (100 µg) is given		
Ketamine	For use in both pediatric and adult patients where sedation, analgesia and amnesia are required	Intravenous: The minimum dose at which dissociative state can be reliably achieved is 1.5 mg/kg Note: Acceptable to start at 0.5 mg/kg and titrate until dissociative state has been achieved Additional incremental dosing: 0.5–1 mg/kg to prolong sedation Intramuscular: The minimum dose at which the dissociative state can be reliably achieved is 4–5 mg/kg intramuscularly	Emergence phenomena: Vomiting, dysphoric reactions, disequilibrium, skin reaction, respiratory depression (rare), laryngospasm	Unique form of procedural sedation, called dissociative sedation, whereby visual, auditory and tactile sensory input is modulated in such a way that the usual higher cortical processing and response is blunted resulting in trance-like, cataleptic or fugue state characterized by blank stare with nystagmus

agents are used, at least two hours should have elapsed since the last use of these agents to prevent the possibility of re-sedation.

Patients should be provided with written, understandable discharge instructions that include possible post-procedure complications and actions to be taken if present. They should be discharged accompanied by a reliable (adult) escort who can understand the discharge instructions and monitor the patient for post-procedure complications. Patients may not drive and it is recommended that they refrain from making important decisions for 24 hours.

SUGGESTED READINGS

1. Aldrete J. A post-anesthetic recovery score. Anesth Analg. 1970;49:924.
2. Bassett K. Propofol for procedural sedation in children in the emergency department. Ann Emerg Med. 2003;42:773-82.
3. Chudnofsky C, et al. Sedation and analgesia for procedures. In: Rosen P, et al. (Ed). Emergency Medicine: Concepts and Clinical Practices, 6th edition. St Louis, MO. Mosby; 2006. pp. 2938-955.
4. Deitch K. The utility of supplemental oxygen during emergency department procedural sedation and analgesia with midazolam and fentanyl: A randomized, controlled trial. Ann Emerg Med. 2007;49(1):1-8.
5. Di Liddo L. Etomidate versus midazolam for procedural sedation in pediatric outpatients: a randomized controlled trial. Ann Emerg Med. 2006;48(4):433-40.
6. Ducharme J. Procedural sedation in the ED: How, when and which agents to choose. Emerg Med Pract. 2000;2(6):1-20.
7. Frank R. Procedural sedation in adults. UpToDate. 2011
8. Goodwin SA. Clinical policy: Procedural sedation and analgesia in the emergency department. Ann Emerg Med. 2005;45:177-96.
9. Goodwin SA. Clinical policy: Procedural sedation and analgesia in the emergency department. Ann Emerg Med. 2005;45:177-96.
10. Graff K. Conscious sedation for pediatric orthopedic procedures. Pediatric Emergency Care. 1996;12(1):31-5.
11. Green S. Should capnographic monitoring be standard practice during emergency department procedural sedation and analgesia? Pro and Con. Ann Emerg Med. 2010;55(3):265-7.
12. Green SM. Clinical practice guideline for emergency department ketamine dissociative sedation in children. Ann Emerg Med. 2004;44:460-71.
13. Green SM. Predictors of airway and respiratory adverse events with ketamine sedation in the emergency department: An individual-patient data meta-analysis of 8282 children. Ann Emerg Med. 2009;54:158-68.

14. Green SM. Predictors of emesis and recovery agitation with emergency department ketamine sedation: An individual-patient data meta-analysis of 8282 children. Ann Emerg Med. 2009;54:171-80.

15. Gross J. Practice guidelines for sedation and analgesia by non-anesthesiologists. Anesth. 2002;96(4):1004-17.

16. Guenther E. Propofol sedation by emergency physicians for elective pediatric outpatient procedures. Ann Emerg Med. 2003;42:783-91.

17. Jagoda A. ACEP: Clinical policy for procedural sedation and analgesia in the emergency department. Ann Emerg Med. 1998;31(5):663-77.

18. Kennedy R. Comparison of fentanyl/midazolam with ketamine/midazolam for pediatric orthopedic emergencies. Pediatrics. 1998;102(4):956-63.

19. Levitan R. Limitations of difficult airway prediction in emergency department intubated patients. Ann Emerg Med. 2004;44:307-13.

20. Mallampati SR. A clinical sign to predict difficult intubation. A prospective study. Canadian Anasthetists' Society Journal. 1985;32:429-34.

21. Miner J. Clinical practice advisory: Emergency department procedural sedation with propofol. Ann Emerg Med. 2007;50:182-7.

22. Miner J. Randomized clinical trial of etomidate versus propofol for procedural sedation in the emergency department. Ann Emerg Med. 2007;49(1):15-22.

23. Pena B. Adverse events of procedural sedation and analgesia in a pediatric emergency department. Ann Emerg Med. 1999;34(4):483-91.

24. Ramsay M. Controlled sedation with alphaxalone-alphadolone. Br Med J. 1974;2:656-9.

25. Ruth W. Intravenous etomidate for procedural sedation in emergency department patients. Acad Emerg Med. 2001;8:13-18.

26. Schenarts C. Adrenocortical dysfunction following etomidate induction in emergency medicine patients. Acad Emerg Med. 2001;8(1):1-7.

27. Sener S. Ketamine with and without midazolam for emergency department sedation in adults: A randomized controlled trial. Ann Emerg Med. 2011;57(2):109-114.

28. Steward J. A simplified scoring system for the post-operative recovery room. Canad Anaesth Soc J. 1975;22(1):111-3.

29. Taylor D. Propofol versus midazolam/fentanyl for reduction of anterior shoulder dislocation. Acad Emerg Med. 2005;12(1):13-19.

30. Vinson, D. Etomidate for Procedural Sedation in Emergency Medicine. Ann Emerg Med. 2002;39(6):592-8.

31. White PF. Ketamine, its pharmacology and therapeutic uses. Anesthesiology. 1982;56:119-36.

32. Willman E. A prospective evaluation of "ketofol" (ketamine/propofol combination) for procedural sedation and analgesia in the emergency department. Ann Emerg Med. 2007;49(1):23-30.

33. Willoughby RE. Survival after treatment of rabies with induction of coma. NEJM. 2005;352:2508-14.

Index

Page numbers followed by *f* refers to figure.